Edited by E.I. Hernández-Jiménez, E.M. Rakhanskaya

SENSITIVE SKIN
IN COSMETIC DERMATOLOGY
& SKINCARE PRACTICE

Cosmetics & Medicine
Publishing

Author/Editor:
Elena I. Hernández-Jiménez, *Ph.D.*

Editor:
Ekaterina M. Rakhanskaya, *M.D.* Neurologist, radiation safety specialist

Contributors:
Vera I. Albanova, *M.D., Ph.D., Prof.* Dermatologist
Aida G. Gadzhigoroeva, *M.D., Ph.D.* Dermatologist, trichologist
Natalia N. Nikolaeva, *M.D., Ph.D.* Dermatologist, psychologist
Yulia Y. Romanova, *M.D.* Dermatologist, trichologist

SENSITIVE SKIN IN THE COSMETIC DERMATOLOGY AND SKINCARE PRACTICE

Patients with sensitive skin often pose a problem for skincare specialists. First, as their complaints are often subjective — burning, itching, tightness, and tingling, which cannot be seen with the naked eye — it is not always clear what to work with and how to diagnose and evaluate the therapy outcomes. Second, for many people, skin hypersensitivity is typically initiated by cosmetics, which is the main skincare tool, so skincare practitioners may avoid such clients who likely expect cosmetics used in treatment to only make things worse.

Yet, this is not the case, as the right cosmetic care and treatment can take away the unpleasant symptoms, thereby contributing to a significant improvement in the quality of life for people with sensitive skin.

This book was created to help dermatologists and other skincare professionals better understand this syndrome, allowing them to tailor their correction protocols to each case.

For this purpose, we have gathered as much up-to-date information as possible, given that research in recent years has helped to make significant advances in our understanding of this condition. Why do not all patients with sensitive skin have problems with the skin barrier, even though it was previously considered a "must"? Why is hypersensitivity present even though a reduction in nerve endings is found in many patients? Does the microbiome influence the development of sensitivity symptoms, and what are the dangers of psychological stress? You will find the answers to these and other questions in our new book. This is important knowledge and new nuances presented within these pages will help you build a truly effective therapy.

The main part of the book is devoted to building an effective care strategy for sensitive skin. For this purpose, all complex treatment approaches are considered, from limiting triggers, protection, and cleansing, which are very specific to this condition, to modern therapeutic modalities that affect each of the mechanisms of sensitive skin pathogenesis. As all of them have their own nuances, these will also be discussed in detail.

In addition, the peculiarities of diagnosing this condition and how to distinguish it from other skin pathologies — atopic, allergic, contact dermatitis, and rosacea — are provided. Separate sections are devoted to the problems of skin sensitivity with age-related changes, the possibilities of correcting the symptoms of sensitive scalp, as well as psychological help to patients which can be provided by a skincare specialist. These issues are rarely talked about, but addressing them greatly improves the condition of patients with sensitive skin syndrome.

Given the wealth of information presented in this book, it will be useful to dermatologists and skincare specialists working with individuals experiencing sensitive skin problems, as well as all interested parties. Of course, it will also help people with sensitive skin to evaluate advertising claims in a balanced way and to base their skincare on reliable information.

ISBN 978-1-970196-23-8 (paperback)
ISBN 978-1-970196-45-0 (hardcover)
ISBN 978-1-970196-06-1 (eBook – Adobe PDF)
ISBN 978-1-970196-15-3 (eBook – ePUB)

FirstEditing

English version is edited and certified by the FirstEditing.Com, Inc. (USA).

Author/Editor

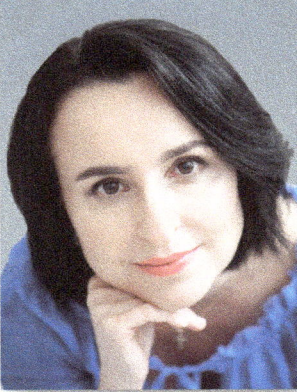

Elena I. Hernández-Jiménez, *Ph.D.*

Biophysicist, scientific journalist

Editor-in-chief of Cosmetics and Medicine Publishing

Chairperson of the Executive Board of the International Society of Applied Corneotherapy (I.A.C.)

Author and co-author of numerous publications in professional magazines, co-author and editor of the book series *Fundamentals of Cosmetic Dermatology & Skincare*, *Cosmetic Dermatology & Skincare Practice*, *Cosmetic Chemistry for Dermatology & Skincare Specialists* and others

Speaker at international conferences, author of training seminars and webinars for professionals in the field of skincare

Professional interests: biology and physiology of the skin, skin permeability, cosmetic chemistry, anti-age medicine, physiotherapy in dermatology and aesthetic medicine, skin analysis and imaging

Table of Contents

PART V
AGE-RELATED CHANGES IN SKIN SENSITIVITY

Abbreviations

ACTH — adrenocorticotropic hormone

AHA — alpha-hydroxy acid

AMP — antimicrobial peptide

ASIC — acid-sensitive ion channels

ATP — adenosine triphosphate

CAMP — cathelicidin antimicrobial peptide

Cer — ceramide

CGRP — calcitonin gene-related peptide

Chol — cholesterol

CNS — central nervous system

CRH — corticotropin-releasing hormone

DNA — deoxyribonucleic acid

EFA — essential fatty acids

FDA — U.S. Food and Drug Administration

FFA — free fatty acids

IBS — irritable bowel syndrome

ICD — International Classification of Diseases

IFSI — International Forum for the Study of Itch

IL — interleukin

INCI — International Nomenclature of Cosmetic Ingredients

KLK5 — kallikrein 5

LLLT — low-level laser (light) therapy

MMP — matrix metalloproteinases

MRI — magnetic resonance imaging

NGF — nerve growth factor

NHE1 — sodium–hydrogen exchanger 1

NMF — natural moisturizing factor

PABA — para-aminobenzoic acid

PACAP — pituitary adenylate cyclase-activating polypeptide

PDT — photodynamic therapy

PG — prostaglandin

PM — particulate matter

PPAR — peroxisome-proliferator-activated receptors

RNA — ribonucleic acid

SP — substance P

SPF — sun protection factor

sPLA2 — secretory phospholipase 2

TCA — trichloracetic acid

TEWL — transepidermal water loss

TLR — Toll-like receptors

TNF — tumor necrosis factor

TRP — transient receptor potential channels

TRPA — transient receptor potential channels, ankyrin subtype

TRPV — transient receptor potential channels, vanilloid subtype

TTPA — test of the type of personality accentuation

UV — ultraviolet

UVA — ultraviolet type A

UVB — ultraviolet type B

VEGF — vascular endothelial growth factor

VIP — vasoactive intestinal peptide

Introduction

Sensitive skin is a complex problem that many skincare specialists must face. The fact is that the complaints of clients with sensitive skin are often subjective and can include severe irritation of the facial skin, burning or tingling after applying cosmetics or using hygiene products, impacts of various external factors, contact with clothing, or even interaction with plain tap water. As they often have no objective clinical signs such as redness, flaking, swelling, or rashes, there is nothing that would be expected in known cases of inflammatory or allergic skin diseases. It is, therefore, not uncommon for these patients to be viewed with some prejudice, but their problem is real. Moreover, it interferes with their ability to live their life to the full. Therefore, a sensitive and competent specialist can significantly improve their condition.

In our new book, we have compiled all relevant information that will help specialists better understand the problem of sensitive skin and choose the optimal management regimen for these patients.

Part I

Etiology
and pathogenesis
of sensitive skin

The concept of "sensitive skin" was introduced by Arthur Kligman and Peter Frosch in 1977 (Frosch P.J., Kligman A.M., 1977). Henry Maibach in 1987 described the symptoms accompanying skin hypersensitivity as "cosmetic intolerance syndrome" (Maibach H.I., 1987). Today, the phrase "sensitive skin" is widely used in everyday life, advertisement, and skincare practice, although it can mean different things:

- Tendency to develop unusual reactions such as tingling, burning, itching, and discomfort in response to cosmetics and exogenous environmental factors (Kligman A.M. et al., 2006).
- Questionable condition characterized by subjective cutaneous hypersensitivity and a significant impact on health-related quality of life (Berardesca E. et al., 2013).
- Condition characterized by a propensity for increased development of dermatitis, inflammatory lesions resulting from skin exposure to damaging factors of chemical, physical, or biological nature (Inamadar A.C., Palit A., 2013).

In 2017, the working group of the International Forum for the Study of Itch (IFSI) defined sensitive skin as **"a syndrome associated with unpleasant sensations (tingling, burning, pain, heat, and itching) in response to stimuli that should not normally provoke such sensations"** (Misery L. et al., 2017). Although this definition is not yet standardized, it is accepted by many specialists worldwide, as it most clearly reflects the essence of the "sensitive skin" phenomenon.

1.1. The epidemic of sensitive skin

If you think that these patients are rare, you are sorely mistaken. Sensitive skin, or sensitive skin syndrome, is a widespread phenomenon.

Although the estimates vary, and are mostly based on self-assessment questionnaires, they are rather alarming and include:

- in the U.S. — 44% of the population (according to documented data), and 60–70% of women and 50–60% of men (according to self-assessment questionnaires (Maibach H.I., 1987; Brenaut E. et al., 2020)
- in the UK — 51% of women and 38% of men (Willis C.M. et al., 2001)
- in India — 36.7% of women and 27.9% of men; with 7.2% of women and 5.1% of men reporting having very sensitive skin (Wang X. et al., 2020)

According to a recent meta-analysis including 26 studies in 18 countries and involving more than 50,000 people, 45% of women and 33% of men (38% in the Americas, 35% in South America, 44% in Europe, and 31% in Asia) have sensitive skin (Chen W. et al., 2020).

Women suffer from high skin sensitivity more often than men, which seems related to a smaller skin thickness, daily use of various cosmetic products, and monthly hormonal fluctuations (Farage M.A., 2010; Chen W. et al., 2020). It is probably due to hormonal fluctuations that skin hypersensitivity in women is more common in premenopausal and older age groups. At the same time, men may be more sensitive to emotional stimuli (Wang X. et al., 2020). However, it is hypothesized that, owing to the increased production and use of a variety of hygiene and cosmetic products for men, as well as the frequency of male visits to cosmetic facilities, gender-specific skin sensitivity rates will likely equalize.

It is not only the skin of the face that can be hypersensitive. As this issue tends to be correlated with the extent of exposure to aggressive factors, other areas of the body are involved in 70% of cases (Saint-Martory C. et al., 2008):

- in 58% — hands
- in 36% — scalp
- in 34% — feet
- in 27% — neck
- in 23% — torso
- in 21% — back
- In 61% — whole body

It should also be noted that the direct correlation between photo-type and race is controversial. Although it was previously thought that skin hypersensitivity was more common in fair-skinned individuals, it is also a problem that affects people with darker phototypes, but their complaints may differ (Foster M.W., Sharp R.R., 2002; Farage M.A., Maibach H.I., 2010). That said, it is interesting that more than 50% of dark-skinned women living in the United States consider their skin to be sensitive (some studies have even found them to be more sensitive than light-skinned women), but dark-skinned women living in Africa have a lower rate of skin sensitivity (Brenaut E. et al., 2020). In general, it can be assumed that skin sensitivity is a problem that predominantly affects those living in developed countries. To some extent, this may explain the "sensitive skin epidemic" — the term used to indicate rapid increase in the number of cases. The reason for this upward trend may be the wide availability of cosmetic and hygienic products, the pollution of megacities, and the stressful rhythm of life in them, i.e., the excess of trigger factors for sensitive skin, which we will discuss further.

1.2. Triggers of sensitive skin syndrome

Sensitive skin can be susceptible to many irritating factors. However, the immediate "enemies" are individualized for each specific patient and can be broadly divided into three groups:

- **Direct contact with the skin** — insufficiently skin-friendly substances in cosmetics, hard water, and certain fabrics can cause itching, tingling, tightness, and/or redness
- **External factors** — heat, cold, or rapid temperature changes, wind, insolation, and dust can cause tingling, burning, redness, and hot flushes
- **Vascular factors** — with increased permeability of the vascular wall (due to ambient temperature fluctuations, ingestion of a number of spices, and alcohol consumption, as well as disruption of the microcirculation regulation mechanisms in some diseases, such as rosacea), hot flushes, redness, and hypersensitivity to heat will be the leading symptoms

In most patients, symptoms appear within one hour of exposure to triggers and may persist for several minutes or even hours (Misery L., 2017).

In a recent meta-analysis, Brenaut E. et al. (2020) examined the contribution of different triggers (provoking factors) to the development of sensitive skin. To this end, the authors reviewed all studies on sensitive skin triggers posted in PubMed — the largest database of medical and biological publications — between 1990 and 2018. Thirteen papers related to studies involving 20,486 participants that completed questionnaires about sensitive skin triggers during face-to-face and telephone interviews, or internet surveys were included in the final analysis. The results, defined as an odds ratio — the probability of skin sensitivity symptoms in response to a trigger in people with sensitive skin relative to the odds of the same phenomenon in a control group of individuals with healthy skin — are presented in **Table I-1-1**.

Table I-1-1. Triggers for sensitive skin, based on the data derived from surveys (Brenaut E. et al., 2020)

TRIGGER FACTOR	ODDS RATIO	95% CI*
Cosmetic products	7.12	3.98–12.72
Humid air	3.83	2.48–5.91
Air conditioning	3.60	2.11–6.14
Temperature changes	3.53	2.69–4.63
Hot temperature	3.50	2.56–4.77
Contact with water	3.46	2.82–4.25
Environmental pollutants	3.18	2.37–4.27
Dry air	3.04	2.22–4.16
Cold	2.73	1.94–3.84
Wind	2.33	1.69–3.22
Sun	1.81	1.61–2.04
Emotions	1.77	1.44–2.17

* CI — confidence interval.

As the findings reported in **Table I-1-1** show, cosmetics are the main factor that patients attribute to the onset of their skin sensitivity symptoms. They also concur with the results yielded by a study involving 869 women, as a part of which a variety of cosmetic and hygiene products were tested to compare their "irritant" potential in people with sensitive and healthy skin (Richters R.J.H. et al., 2017). The results are presented in **Table I-1-2**.

Table I-1-2. Frequency of skin sensitivity symptoms in response to the use of cosmetic and hygiene products among 869 women with sensitive and healthy (non-sensitive) skin (Richters R.J.H. et al., 2017)

PRODUCT	SENSITIVE SKIN	HEALTHY SKIN
Soap	72%	24%
Powdery (tightening) facial products	69%	27%
Facial cleansers	68%	21%
Lotions and body moisturizers	62%	13%
Products with fragrances	61%	17%
Facial cosmetics	60%	14%
Facial moisturizers and lotions	60%	17%
Deodorants	51%	21%
Perfume	48%	15%
Antiperspirants	48%	19%
Sun protection agents	46%	13%
Hair dyes	42%	20%
Fabric softeners	38%	11%
Hair styling products (sprays, gels, mousses)	31%	12%
Shampoos	30%	11%

Interestingly, despite the leading position of cosmetic products in provoking symptoms of sensitive skin, the role of hair coloring products was investigated (and confirmed) in only one study (Bernard A. et al., 2016). As the personal experience of many practitioners suggests that such a problem does exist, we will consider sensitive scalp in detail in a separate section.

In addition to the trigger factors mentioned above, the interviewees noted contact with clothing (Richters R.J.H. et al., 2017). Current or prior smoking also slightly increased the risk of skin sensitization, presumably due to generally negative effects on the skin barrier (Falcone D. et al., 2017a).

However, we should again draw attention to the fact that the relationship between all these factors and skin sensitivity was assessed only from the patients' perspective. For more precise data, it is necessary to conduct objective studies.

Hormonal fluctuations, including those associated with the menstrual cycle, can also increase skin sensitivity. In a study involving 278 women, about 42% of the sample reported increased skin sensitivity just before and during their menstrual cycle. The authors also attributed this finding to a deterioration in barrier function due to low estrogen levels during menstruation. Low estrogen levels may also partially contribute to the higher prevalence of sensitive skin among peri- and postmenopausal women (Falcone D. et al., 2017b).

It is important to note that many dermatologic diseases may be accompanied by increased skin sensitivity, such as atopic dermatitis, acne, and psoriasis. Such patients face problems with sensitive skin about 2.5 times more often than healthy people (Falcone D. et al., 2017b). However, the problem of sensitive skin is particularly pronounced in individuals suffering from rosacea.

1.3. How the skin senses: cutaneous sensory receptors

Before turning to the pathophysiologic mechanisms of skin hypersensitivity, let us briefly address how skin sensitivity is formed.

Our skin is a huge receptor field sensitive to various external signals (**Fig. I-1-1**). The skin is innervated by the peripheral nervous system from the ganglia of the spinal cord and trigeminal nerve. Some fibers (of the subepidermal plexus) cross the dermo-epidermal junction and enter the epidermis (so-called intra-epidermal fibers).

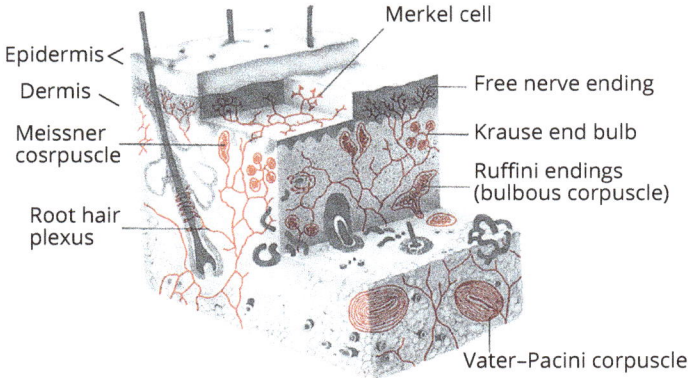

Figure I-1-1. Cutaneous receptors and their functions

RECEPTOR / FUNCTION		RECEPTOR / FUNCTION	
Free nerve endings	Free nerve endings are the most common nerve endings in skin, and they extend into the middle of the epidermis. Free nerve endings are sensitive to painful stimuli, to hot and cold, and to light touch.	Krause end bulbs	They are on the surface and are very sensitive to low temperatures, so they "feel" the cold.
Meissner corpuscle	Meissner corpuscles are ellipsoid mechanoreceptors located superficially within the dermal papillae at a depth of approximately 150 μm. Sensitive to light touch, numerous on the pads of the fingers and tip of the tongue. Allow to determine the size of the objects.	Merkel cell	Merkel cells are connected to the nerve endings in the skin that are responsible for the sense of touch. They are found in particularly sensitive areas of the skin (e.g., the lips) and are surrounded by the thinnest endings of the sensory nerves.
Vater–Pacini corpuscle	Vater–Pacini corpuscle is one of the four major types of mechanoreceptors located in the deepest part of the dermis. Most of these corpuscles respond only to sudden disturbances and are especially sensitive to vibration of few hundreds of Hz. The vibrational role may be used for detecting surface texture, e.g., rough vs. smooth. A few are also sensitive to quasi-static or low frequency pressure stimuli.	Ruffini endings (bulbous corpuscle)	Ruffini endings are small, spindle-shaped, slowly adapting receptors found throughout the dermis, subcutaneous tissue, and some connective tissues. They are situated deeper than Krause's end bulbs and, being sensitive to elevated temperatures, they perceive heat. However, as there are fewer of these corpuscles, the sensation of heat is perceived more slowly than the sensation of cold, so it is easy to get sunburned if care is not taken.

The receptors are the endings of nerve fibers, which differ in structure and function. The cutaneous receptors (exteroceptors) include:

- **Free nerve endings** — located in the epidermis or around the base of the hair in the dermal layer (register hair movement)
- **Encapsulated receptors** — surrounded by a connective tissue sheath **(Meissner corpuscles, Vater–Pachini corpuscles, Ruffini endings, and Krause end bulbs)**, and lie at different depths in the dermal layer
- **Merkel cells (Merkel disks)** — independent cells (not nerve endings) located in the epidermis

On a functional basis, the following groups of receptors can be recognized:

- **Thermoreceptors** that sense changes in temperature
- **Mechanoreceptors** that register skin touch, squeezing, and vibration
- **Nociceptors** that respond to painful stimuli

Touch receptors dominate the human skin. Apparently, each individual receptor perceives a specific tactile sensation, but when the skin is exposed to different mechanical stimuli, several types of receptors react simultaneously.

Cutaneous sensitivity is multimodal. For the perception of touch (pressure, vibration, and texture), there are four types of specialized nerve structures in the skin: Meissner's corpuscles, Vater–Pacini, Ruffini, and Merkel's discs (**Fig. I-1-2**). They belong to mechanoreceptors with a low threshold of sensitivity. Thus, Meissner's and Vater–Pacini corpuscles react only to the beginning and end of a mechanical stimulus, while Merkel's disks and Ruffini's corpuscles react to a constantly acting stimulus. Each specialized structure has a so-called receptive field — an area with receptors that, when exposed to a certain stimulus, leads to a change in the neuron's excitation. The receptive field is smaller in Meissner's corpuscles and Merkel's disks located at the basal membrane of the epidermis, i.e., closer to the skin surface, and is larger in Ruffini's and Vater–Pacini corpuscles located deeper in the dermis. The signals received from the skin surface are transmitted via myelinated Aδ nerve fibers to the central nervous system (CNS).

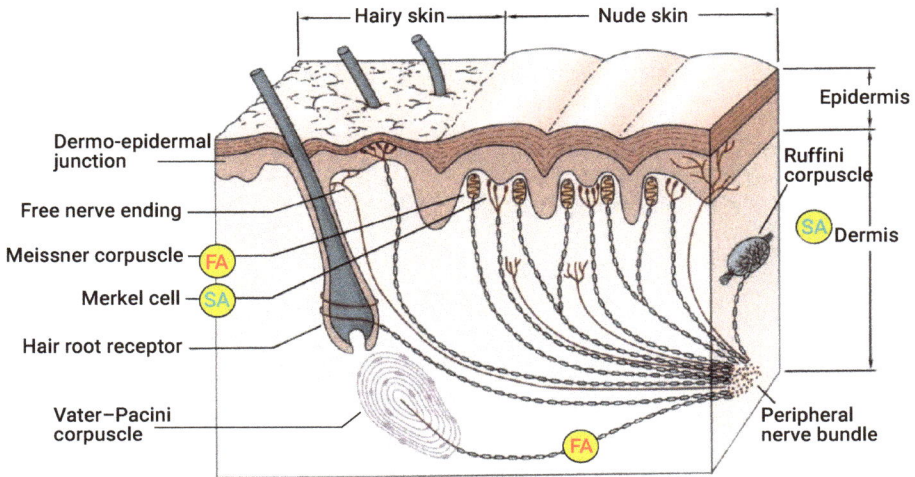

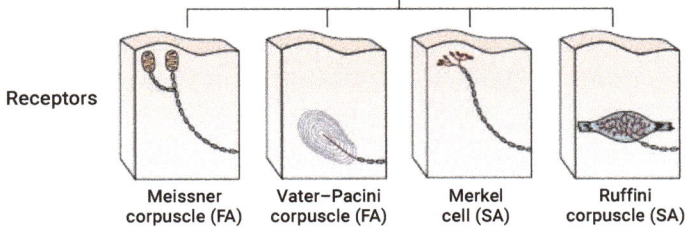

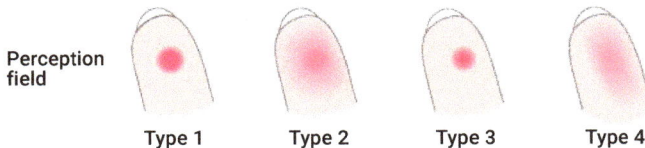

Figure I-1-2. Localization of the cutaneous receptors

Abbreviations: FA — fast adapting fibers; SA — slow adapting fibers

How are we aware of tactile stimuli? In the CNS, special structures control touch, recognition, attention, and emotion and combine the signals received with signals from other systems (vision, olfaction). As a result, touch can be realized in the CNS as a wide range of sensations — soft, hard, rough, smooth, wet, sticky, prickly, cool, warm, heavy, pleasant, and unpleasant — of varying intensity.

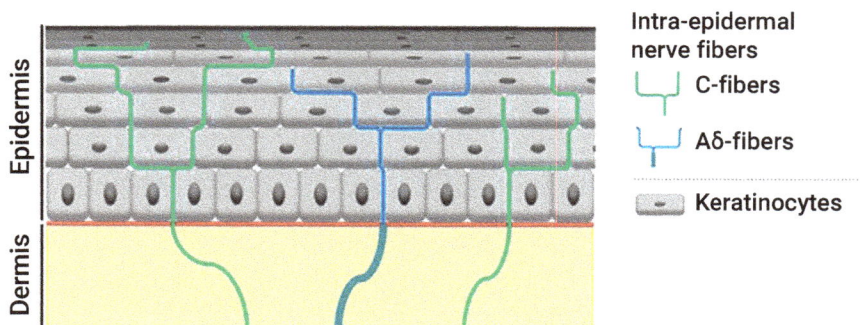

Figure I-1-3. Intra-epidermal nerve fibers
(adapted from Talagas M., Misery L., 2019)

Intra-epidermal nerve fibers, classified as C- and Aδ-fibers, unmyelinated and thickly myelinated, respectively, are conventionally described as the exclusive sensors for temperature, pain, and itch. Aδ-fibers lose their myelin sheath when crossing the basement membrane.

As there are no specialized structures for the perception of temperature and pain (including irritation, pinching, burning, searing, pricking, and the pain itself), signals are transmitted via free nerve endings — myelinated (Aδ) and unmyelinated C-nerve fibers (**Fig. I-1-3**). Both types of fibers penetrate the basal membrane of the epidermis, and their branched nerve endings extend into the epidermis, in close contact with keratinocytes. The termination of each fiber forms a sensitive spot for cold or warmth detection. The spots are unevenly distributed in different body parts: on the lips, there are 15–25 cold spots/cm², the fingers contain 3–5 spots/cm², while the torso only has 1 spot/cm². There are 3–10 times fewer sensitive warmth spots than cold ones. The most sensitive skin area is the face, where the sensitivity also varies, being the highest in the nasolabial fold, followed by malar eminence, chin, and forehead, and is the lowest in the upper lip.

Each nerve fiber serves a circumference of approximately 1 mm in diameter. As well as from specialized nerve structures, the signal is carried by free nerve endings (afferent) through the spinal cord to the CNS.

In addition to their perceptive function, receptors release various biologically active substances into the surrounding extracellular space, which serve as mediators and participate in local extracellular communication processes. Thus, under prolonged strong stimulation, free nerve endings release substance P (SP) and calcitonin gene-related peptide (CGRP), which cause vascular dilation and increase the permeability of the vascular wall.

Here, as well as in the perception of various types of stimuli by free nerve endings, special receptors, particularly cation channels with transient receptor potential (TRP), play a role. This is a large family of transmembrane receptors that regulate permeability to cations, mainly Ca^{2+} and Mg^{2+}, and are located both in the free nerve endings of sensitive neurons and in keratinocytes, fibroblasts, blood vessels, immune system cells, and mast cells, as well as in many other tissues of the body, including the intestine (**Fig. I-1-4**). These channels are activated by physical and chemical factors, and their pathologic or enhanced stimulation is possible (Caterina M.J. et al., 2016; Emir T.L.R., 2017).

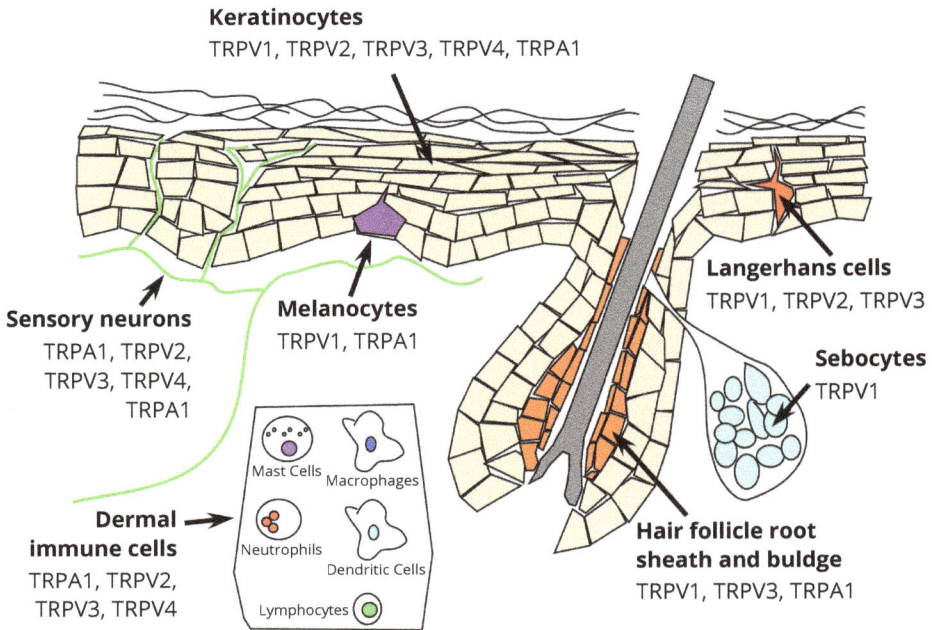

Keratinocytes
TRPV1, TRPV2, TRPV3, TRPV4, TRPA1

Sensory neurons
TRPA1, TRPV2,
TRPV3, TRPV4,
TRPA1

Melanocytes
TRPV1, TRPA1

Langerhans cells
TRPV1, TRPV2, TRPV3

Sebocytes
TRPV1

Mast Cells Macrophages

**Dermal
immune cells**
TRPA1, TRPV2,
TRPV3, TRPV4

Neutrophils

Dendritic Cells

Lymphocytes

**Hair follicle root
sheath and buldge**
TRPV1, TRPV3, TRPA1

Figure I-1-4. TRPV and TRPA channels in the skin
(adapted from Caterina M.J., 2014)

Several types of TRP are known, the main ones being (Bouvier V. et al., 2018; Storozhuk M.V., Zholos A.V., 2018):

- TRP of the vaniloid sybtype 1 (TRPV1) which is activated by capsaicin, phorbol esters, heat, pH below 7 (acidic values), and ultraviolet light
- TRPV3 which is stimulated by heat and camphor
- TRPV4 which responds to heat, mechanical pressure, hypoosmolar stress, and phorbol ester derivatives
- TRPV8 which is triggered by cold and menthol
- TRP of the ankyrin subtype 1 (TRPA1) which is activated by mustard oil, cold, and various chemical components

When they are excited, the corresponding sensations (hot, cold, burning, pain) occur, and inflammatory processes are triggered. This is due to the release of vasoactive neuropeptides such as SP and CGRP, vasoactive intestinal peptide (VIP), and pituitary adenylate cyclase-activating polypeptide (PACAP). Substance P is involved in the local regulation of blood flow and induces mast cell degranulation, leading to increased levels of pro-inflammatory cytokines (e.g., IL-1, IL-3, and IL-8), chemokines (e.g., CCL2, CXCL9, CXCL10, CCL5, and CXCL8), tumor necrosis factor alpha (TNFα), and vascular endothelial growth factor (VEGF). These are natural responses to compensate for the effects of stimuli, but they can be excessive, and this is the basis of a process called **neurogenic inflammation** (Aubdool A.A., Brain S.D., 2011; Buddenkotte J., Steinhoff M., 2018).

So far, we have discussed structures that perceive signals from the outside, i.e., afferent structures. Through the sympathetic nervous system, the same sensitive fibers pass efferent signals. The sympathetic nervous system regulates the tone of blood vessels (vasoconstrictor fibers), the activity of skin gland secretion (motor fibers), and involuntary skin muscles (pilomotor fibers). The major neurotransmitters are noradrenaline, adrenaline, and acetylcholine. Transmission of efferent nerve impulses affects the production of histamine and other biologically active substances by mast cells as a result of scratching and other reactions.

Research conducted in recent years has demonstrated that the skin interacts with the CNS and the brain directly, and this interaction is constant, bidirectional, and very intense. Information from the receptors goes to the CNS, where it is processed and analyzed. From there, the body receives a command on how to react to the signal.

1.4. Pathogenesis of the sensitive skin

It should be said at the outset that there is still no complete picture of the sensitive skin syndrome pathogenesis. However, the discoveries made in recent years have helped to make significant progress in this direction, and it seems that now we already have some semblance of unity in this picture.

The fact is that, for a long time, two main hypotheses of the formation of skin sensitivity syndrome have predominated — violation of the barrier function of the skin and hypersensitivity of nerve fibers. It is known that increased skin permeability facilitates access to various kinds of stimuli to sensory nerves. However, studies have shown that impaired barrier function is not observed in all patients with sensitive skin symptoms, and the number of nerve fibers in their skin is often decreased rather than increased. Therefore, although related to each other, these two hypotheses do not explain all variants of pathology and not in all cases. Let us consider them and the discoveries that have been made recently.

1.4.1. Skin barrier in the sensitive skin

As we have mentioned above, one of the main hypotheses associated with the formation of sensitive skin syndrome is the violation of the integrity of the skin barrier. It is the broken skin barrier that facilitates access of foreign agents to sensitive skin structures, which causes unpleasant sensations from seemingly ordinary actions.

Disruption of the epidermal barrier is expected mainly in persons suffering from skin diseases such as atopic dermatitis, xerosis, acne, or rosacea. In addition, external aggressive influences, whether associated with the prescription of certain drugs or cosmetic procedures, are also involved in disrupting the epidermal barrier. Examples of medications are benzoyl peroxide, azelaic acid, and retinoids for acne and rosacea. Examples of cosmetic procedures are microneedling, microdermabrasion, chemical peeling, and laser treatments. Simple everyday hygiene and cosmetic procedures, ultraviolet (UV) radiation, environmental pollutants, etc., can also cause damage. All this leads to greater skin barrier permeability, whereby water easily leaves it, and foreign substances penetrate, including the structures that contribute to skin sensitivity.

When water deficiency occurs, the corneocytes shrivel and deform, leading to the sensation of skin tightness and alteration of enzyme activity. Enzymes cannot function normally under moisture-deficient conditions, and the processes of corneodesmosome destruction and desquamation are disturbed (Farage M.A., Maibach H.I., 2010).

Disruption or, more precisely, destruction of the epidermal barrier in individuals suffering from sensitive skin is characterized by thinning of the epidermis, changes in the composition of extracellular lipids, malformed cornified envelopes, prematurely lost corneodesmosomes, impaired innate immunity, high level of neurotransmitters in the skin, overexpression of TRPV1, and high nerve growth factor (NGF) level (Angelova-Fischer I., 2016; Angelova-Fischer I. et al., 2018; Misery L., 2017; Jiang B. et al., 2019; Talagas M. et al., 2018).

The state of the microcirculatory network is closely related to the epidermal barrier disruption. In sensitive skin, the density of vessels that tend to form a dense network and branching is significantly higher than in healthy skin (Jiang W.C. et al., 2020). This feature has served as a basis to propose dermatoscopy and confocal laser microscopy as diagnostic tools for the sensitive skin syndrome (Zha W.F. et al., 2012).

However, accelerated transepidermal water loss (TEWL) and dry skin, phenomena that are indicative of impaired skin barrier integrity, are not present in all individuals with sensitive skin. In some patients, there is no change in epidermal thickness, no increase in TEWL, and no imbalance in skin lipids (Richters R.J.H. et al., 2017). Sensitive skin syndrome can also be observed in people with oily skin (Hong J.Y. et al., 2020). Based on these inconsistencies, many experts have concluded that a sensory component still plays a primary role in the emergence of sensitive skin syndrome.

1.4.2. Sensory alterations in the sensitive skin

Since itching is one of the main symptoms of sensitive skin, let us briefly review this phenomenon before turning to the peculiarities of the functioning of the sensory systems of sensitive skin.

How the sensation of itching is formed

Itching is mainly caused by histamine secreted by mast cells. Histamine acts on the free nerve endings pervading the dermis and epidermis, which have special histamine receptors that are so sensitive that they can be activated even by minor changes in the extracellular environment, e.g., pH changes or slight mechanical impacts.

The sensation of itching is transmitted to the brain by slow-conducting unmyelinated nerve fibers named C-fibers (Sann H., Pierau F.K., 1998). These fibers transmit the sensation of warmth and dull and aching pain, tingling, and burning. Acute pain is transmitted by faster myelinated Aδ-fibers, which originate from receptors at the epidermis–dermis interface (**Fig. I-1-5**). The free nerve endings of C-fibers and pain A-receptors are called nociceptors (from Latin *nocere* — to damage). Interestingly, the sensations of itching and pain are provided by different response systems. If the epidermis (in which the free nerve endings are located) is removed, itching cannot be induced. However, pain sensitivity is preserved. As severe pain is the antagonist of itching, an intense pain stimulus can suppress itching accompanying some skin diseases for several months.

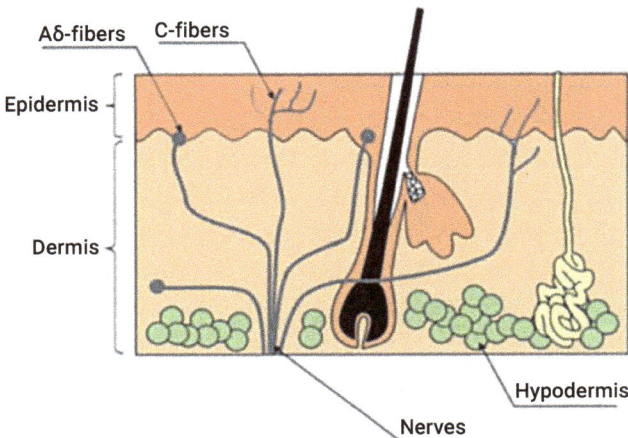

Figure I-1-5. Nociceptors of the skin

The free nerve endings in the epidermis are the first sentinel post of the skin. They allow a person or animal to feel a light touch. Itching, which some people experience when in contact with wool or synthetic fabrics, is also a result of C-receptor irritation. The natural response to itching is scratching, a reflex hand movement that removes the irritant.

The nerve impulse travels along the C-fiber to interneurons in the posterior horns of the spinal cord. Here, it switches to the afferent (motor) nerve fiber responsible for the scratching reflex. Another nerve fiber sends the impulse to the cerebral cortex (**Fig. I-1-6**). If the irritation does not stop or exceeds a certain threshold value,

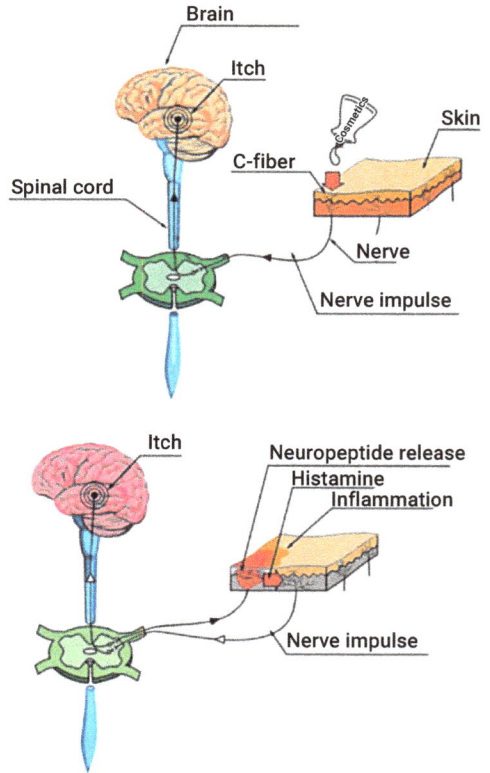

Figure I-1-6. Pathogenesis of neurogenic inflammation

the interneurons of the spinal cord send a reverse (retrograde) impulse to the skin via the C-fiber. This is where the most interesting part begins.

The phenomenon of neurogenic inflammation

The role of C-fibers is not limited to the perception and transmission of information. Having received a retrograde impulse from the spinal cord, they begin to secrete various biologically active substances, the main of which is SP, a neuropeptide consisting of 11 amino acids. Receptors for SP are present in mast cells, lymphocytes, macrophages, sebocytes, and blood vessel cells. Substance P causes degranulation of mast cells, resulting in the release of histamine and other inflammatory mediators

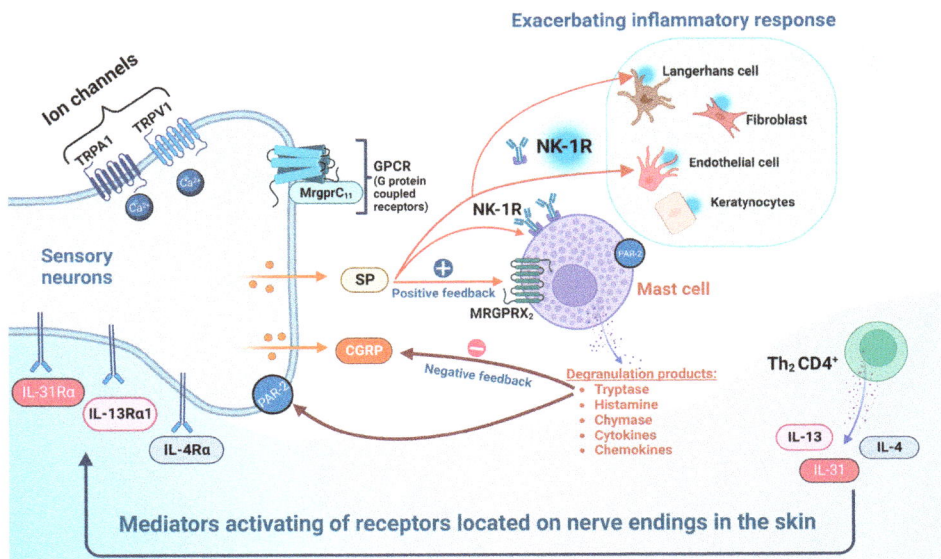

Figure I-1-7. Cellular mechanisms of neurogenic inflammation (adapted from Marek-Jozefowicz L. et al., 2023)

into the extracellular space, activation of macrophages (which also begin to secrete various mediators), dilation of blood vessels, and release of lymphocytes from blood vessels into tissues (**Fig. I-1-7**). In other words, a **full-fledged inflammatory reaction unfolds, the conductors and performers of which are always the cells of the immune system, regardless of the nature of the initial stimulus.**

At this stage, there is also a sensation of itching, now caused by histamine acting on the free nerve endings. It should be noted that mechanical irritation of the free nerve endings during scratching can cause a second wave of excitation along the C-fibers. This can result in a vicious circle: itching — scratching — itching.

The fact that the nervous system plays a significant role in the development of inflammation arising in response to chemical stimuli explains well the nature of the sensory response. Depending on the strength and duration of the irritant stimulus, the skin reaction may be limited to itching (burning, tingling, etc.), or this response may be accompanied by skin reddening and swelling.

Peculiarities of the skin sensory mechanisms involved in the skin sensitivity syndrome

Available evidence indicates that people with sensitive skin have an increased number of TRPV1 receptors which are also activated by capsaicin, phorbol esters, heat exposure, low pH, UV light, and acid-sensitive ion channels (ASICs), including ASIC3 (Kim E.J. et al., 2015).

Moreover, despite the initial assumptions that people with sensitive skin have an increased number of free nerve endings, this is not always the case, as some patients exhibit a decrease in the density of intra-epidermal nerve fibers, mainly C-fibers (Misery L., 2017). However, they also exhibit hypersensitivity (or a decrease in the threshold of sensitivity) of the remaining nerve endings (Misery L., 2017; Huet F. et al., 2018).

Studying the brain response to lactic acid exposure of facial skin using functional magnetic resonance imaging (MRI) brings another interesting confirmation of the neuropathic changes involved in the sensitive skin syndrome. In particular, in people who do not claim to have hypersensitive skin, in response to the discomfort induced by lactic acid application, there is activation of sensorimotor cortical areas on the side opposite to the application, as well as bilateral excitation in the frontal-parietal areas. Conversely, in individuals that report skin hypersensitivity, activation of sensorimotor cortical zones on the side where the product is applied is noted first, and is followed by bilateral excitation of somatosensory zones (Querleux B. et al., 2008). From these observations, we can conclude that the CNS and cortex in people with sensitive skin react differently to stimulation by irritants relative to those of healthy people.

The discrepancy between the richness of sensory symptoms and the reduced density of intra-epidermal nerve fibers seems paradoxical. But everything becomes clear once we take keratinocytes into account. It turns out that their role in the development of sensitive skin syndrome may extend far beyond the construction of the epidermal barrier (Talagas M. et al., 2018). That keratinocytes host many TRP receptors has been known for a relatively long time. Still, recent studies have demonstrated that they may also act as primary nociceptive receptors in addition to sensory neurons.

Sensory properties of keratinocytes

Until recently, it was very difficult to determine the contribution of keratinocytes and sensitive neurons to sensory transmission because of their very close connection; in fact, intra-epidermal nerve fibers seem to braid keratinocytes. However, advances in genetic modification of laboratory organisms have helped solve this problem, as scientists were able to selectively activate TRPV1 or TRPV4 in keratinocytes without simultaneous stimulation of neighboring nerve endings.

According to their findings, the application of capsaicin to the skin of mice genetically modified so that their TRPV1 receptors were expressed exclusively in keratinocytes but not in nerves was sufficient to elicit a protective behavioral response and induce expression of the c-fos, a neuronal activation marker in the ipsilateral dorsal horn of the spinal cord (Pang Z. et al., 2015).

It became clear that keratinocytes are able not only to perceive information about stimuli via TRPV1 but also to transmit it to free nerve endings in an "amount" sufficient for the formation of responses and without the participation of TRPV1 on the nerves themselves. These observations confirmed that keratinocytes are essentially full-fledged pain receptors (**Fig. I-1-8A, B**).

Similarly, the role of the TRPV4 receptors expressed by keratinocytes in itch formation was demonstrated through experimental research. In the study conducted by Chen Y. et al. (2016), combing response induced by intradermal injection of itch-inducing histaminergic substances such as histamine and endothelin-1 was significantly reduced in mice with the *Trpv4* gene turned off in keratinocytes compared with wild-type mice. The same results were obtained for selective TRPV4 inhibitors but not for non-histaminergic compounds such as chloroquine (Chen Y. et al., 2016). Interestingly, this study showed that TRPV4 is turned on after histaminergic itch receptors. As in sensory neurons, TRPV4 is associated with itch receptors, possibly to enhance signaling within keratinocytes and thus to optimize sensory perception (**Fig. I-1-8B**). Beyond these chemical stimuli, the contribution of high temperature to itch perception via TRPV4 expression by keratinocytes remains to be determined (**Fig. I-1-8C**).

In addition to the involvement of TRPV4 in the itch formation process described above, recent data also indicate that keratinocyte-expressed

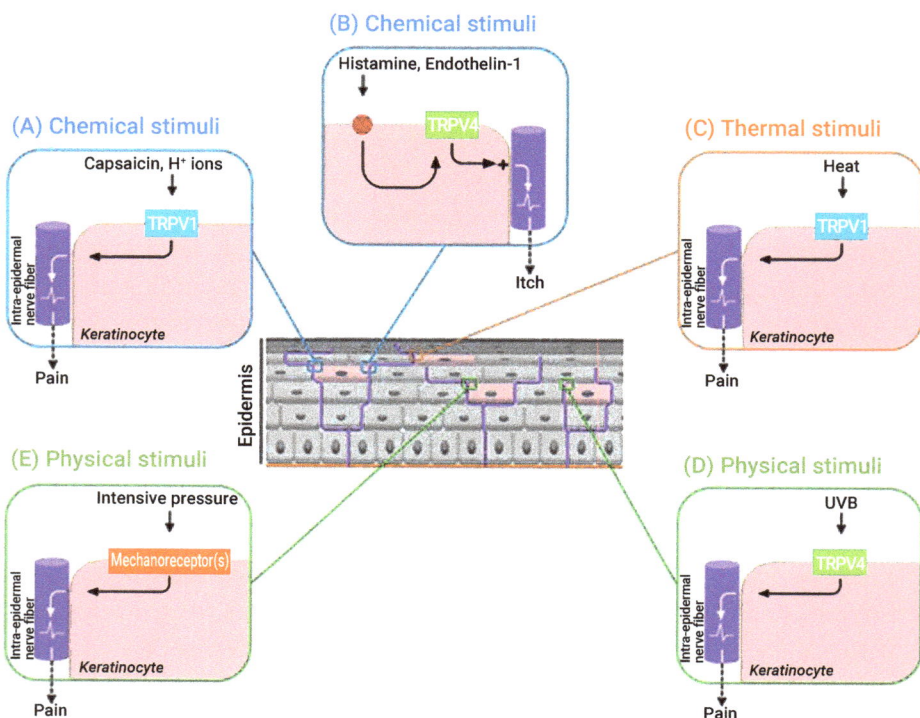

Figure I-1-8. Identified exogenous stimuli and the corresponding keratinocyte sensory receptors triggering pain or itch in mouse models (adaped from Talagas M. et al., 2018)

(A) Chemical stimuli. Capsaicin can induce pain through the activation of keratinocyte-expressed TRPV1. By extension, this process probably involves H+ ions. (B) Chemical stimuli. Histamine and endothelin-1 activate TRPV4 through their respective receptors. Downstream TRPV4 activation induces itch. (C) Thermal stimuli. TRPV1 is also the main transducer of noxious heat. (D) Physical stimuli. UVB activates keratinocyte-expressed TRPV4 to induce pain. (E) Physical stimuli like intense pressure via not yet identified mechanoreceptor(s).

TRPV4 responds to severe UVB exposure by inducing allodynia, pain response to stimuli that do not normally cause it (**Fig. I-1-8D**). These findings indicate that the silencing of *Trpv4* gene in keratinocytes is associated with an attenuated response to harmful thermal and mechanical exposure (**Fig. I-1-8E**). In addition, in response to UVB radiation, the TRPV4 receptor expressed by keratinocytes induces epidermal damage by releasing endothelin-1, a pain- and itch-inducing substance.

Further, endothelin-1 enhances the pro-algetic effect of keratinocyte-expressed TRPV4 via endothelin receptors through autocrine and paracrine pathways (Moore C. et al., 2013).

Consistent with these findings obtained in animal studies, TRPV4 and endothelin-1 immunoreactivity in human skin increase after UV exposure. This helps explain why sunburn and tissue damage in TRPV4-deprived mice is reduced exclusively in epidermal keratinocytes (Talagas M. et al., 2018).

Moreover, optogenetic methods (activation of cellular processes by "introducing" special light-sensitive receptors into cell membranes) are increasingly used to elucidate the role of keratinocytes in response to other stimuli. The obtained results indicate that the keratinocyte "activation" via blue light-sensitive receptors is sufficient to induce an action potential in Aδ- and C-fibers and, ultimately, a protective behavioral response in mice (Baumbauer K.M. et al., 2015). These findings further demonstrate that light stimulation of such modified keratinocytes activates many subtypes of sensory neurons that respond to mechanical and/or thermal stimuli, even if the receptors on keratinocytes that are directly responsible for this action remain unidentified. Consistent with previous data on the keratinocyte expression of TRPV ion channels, these observations emphasize the undeniable influence of keratinocytes on cutaneous sensory perception.

Scientists have also discovered exactly how signal transmission from "excited" keratinocytes to nerve fibers occurs: mechanically stimulated keratinocytes activate sensory neurons through the release of adenosine triphosphate (ATP) (Moehring F. et al., 2018).

Thus, it seems that the role of keratinocytes in the sensitive skin syndrome is not limited to changes in the epidermal barrier and may be related to their sensory properties. This brings together the two hypotheses of hypersensitivity and disrupted skin barrier. In addition, the sensory role of keratinocytes also explains why the number of nerve endings decreases and skin sensitivity increases with age. It is also interesting to note that TRPV1 activation by either capsaicin or temperature exposure delays the barrier repair after damage, whereas the TRPV1 antagonist capsazepine accelerates it. The same is true for TRPV4 (Emir T.L.R., 2017).

Currently, this is the main-stream concept of skin sensitivity syndrome development. It is also interesting because the skin and nervous system originate from the same germinal sheet, the ectoderm (**Fig. I-1-9**). As Dr. Laurent Misery, one of the foremost experts on skin sensitivity, says, "The skin and nervous system are twin brothers who were separated at birth but who are constantly exchanging tidings."

However, as other pathogenetic mechanisms also contribute to the formation of sensitive skin syndrome, they are discussed next.

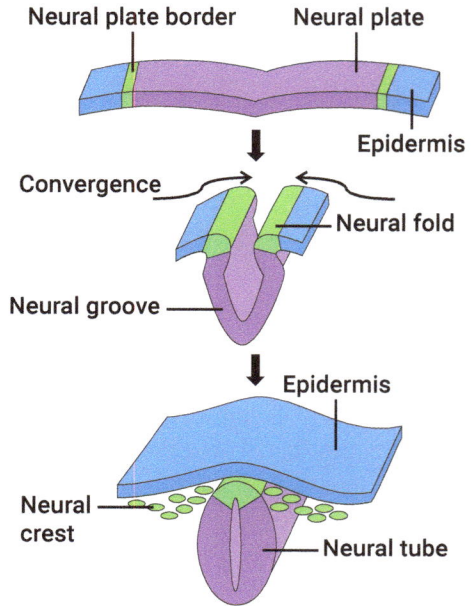

Figure I-1-9. The formation of neural crest during the neurulation process (Image by Wikipedia)

1.4.3. Cell damage

For the body, unplanned damage to the cell membrane is a danger-signaling event, so there is a mechanism built into the cell membranes that allows the body to sense that something is wrong immediately. When the cell membrane is damaged, the molecules from which it is built are broken down. Thus, with the help of the enzyme phospholipase A2, located in the same membrane, phospholipids are broken down, and free fatty acids are released. These free fatty acids are then used to form prostaglandins and other signaling molecules that trigger the inflammation mechanism.

In hypersensitivity, a "storm in a teacup" can occur in the skin. For example, if a surfactant damages the cell membrane, a small number of prostaglandins appear in the skin and a moderate, still invisible, inflammation develops. However, this may be enough to activate C-fibers and cause itching and burning sensations. This hypothesis is supported by the fact that, as a rule, hypersensitive skin reacts to potential irritants (e.g., sodium lauryl sulfate) even at low concentrations. In people with normal skin sensitivity, these substances only cause a reaction when taken in pure form or in high concentrations.

In this case, the fact that skin irritation is invisible does not mean that nothing is going on in the skin. It is just that a person feels something wrong before any external signs emerge.

The mechanisms of hypersensitivity development are now widely studied in cell co-cultures, in which keratinocytes are combined with neurons. In such cell communities, it is possible to perform objective measurements of neuropeptide release and electrical activity of cells, as well as to test the calming effect of various active substances.

1.4.4. Genetic predisposition

Although the genetics of sensitive skin syndrome have not been extensively studied, the obtained findings indicate that it is associated with the increased activity of the *CDH1* gene encoding E-cadherin. E-cadherin is a transmembrane protein involved in the formation of extracellular contacts, maintenance of epidermal integrity, and differentiation of keratinocytes (Kim E.J. et al., 2014).

Yang L. et al. (2017) compared genotyping data from people with sensitive and non-sensitive skin. They identified at least 20 genes that are involved in skin sensitivity, but the role of many of these genes is still unclear. In addition, disorders of various signaling pathways have been identified, including PI3K/Akt (in which E-cadherin is also involved) extracellular matrix receptors, and local adhesion pathway.

1.4.5. Skin blood vessels

Patients with sensitive skin may have vascular hyperreactivity without associated erythema or visible signs of inflammation (Seidenari S. et al., 1998). For example, in the tests with nicotinic acid conducted by Roussaki-Schulze A.V. et al. (2005), Doppler velocimetry showed more significant vasodilation in patients with sensitive skin syndrome than in healthy subjects. There is also evidence for the involvement of histamine (Berardesca E. et al., 2013). Histamine is responsible for the appearance of itching and dilation of the vascular wall. As we have already mentioned, in case of increased vascular wall permeability (due to temperature fluctuations, ingestion of several spices, alcohol consumption, or disturbance of microcirculation regulation mechanisms in some diseases, such as rosacea), the leading symptoms will be hot flushes, redness, and increased sensitivity to heat.

1.4.6. Psychological stress

Exposure to stress factors provokes neuroendocrine, immune, and vascular reactions in the body, affecting all its structures (Misery L., 2017; Talagas M. et al., 2018). The skin is no exception. As stress releases many active substances — both systemically and in the skin itself (**Fig. I-1-10**; **Table I-1-3**) — it disrupts:
- the adherence of the horny scales
- skin immunity (both in the direction of suppression and activation of pathological inflammatory reactions)
- moisture retention capacity of the epidermis
- barrier properties of the skin in general
- regeneration processes
- wound healing, etc.

This manifests not only through changes in skin condition but also leads to the possible induction or exacerbation of dermatologic diseases such as atopic dermatitis, urticaria, psoriasis, rosacea, vitiligo, acne, and alopecia areata.

Current research confirms that stress contributes to the development of both inflammatory and allergic skin diseases and infections, slows wound healing, and causes hair loss. For example, a study focusing on the epidermal barrier function of students during exams and after winter vacation found that stress induced by exams caused an increase in skin permeability and slowed the rate of epidermal barrier repair. These symptoms resolved once students returned from winter break (Bin Saif G.A. et al., 2018). It is also noteworthy that, in patients with a labile nervous system, there is an increase in skin sensitivity under stress, while in calm conditions unpleasant symptoms tend to disappear (Misery L. et al., 2018).

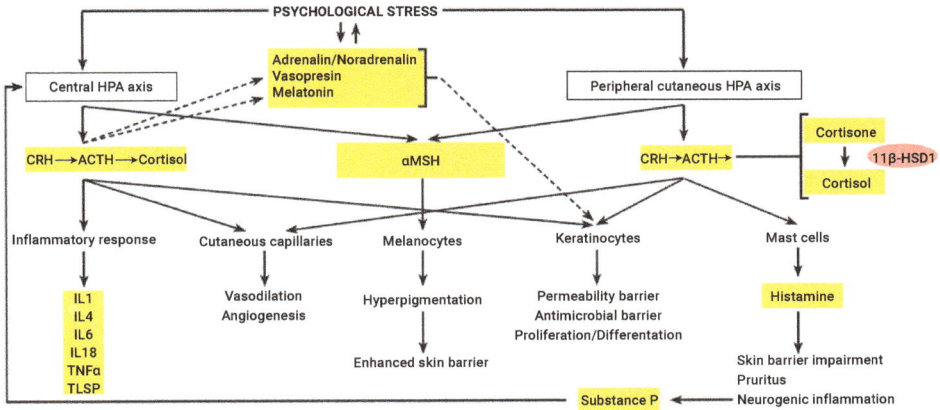

Figure I-1-10. Schematic of the effects of stress on the skin

Table I-1-3. Major stress mediators in the skin (Chen Y., Lyga J., 2014)

STRESS MEDIATOR	SOURCE	EFFECTOR UNIT	FUNCTIONS
Cortico-tropin-releasing hormone (CRH)	• Hypothalamus • Skin: keratinocytes, sebocytes, and mast cells	• The receptor for CRH CRH-R1 is expressed in the epidermis, dermis, and subcutis • CRH-R2 is expressed in hair follicle keratinocytes, and fibroblasts	• Stimulation of ACTH and cortisol production in skin • Cell proliferation • Differentiation • Apoptosis • Inflammation • Angiogenesis
Adreno-cortico-tropic hormone (ACTH)	• Pituitary gland • Skin: melanocytes, epidermal and hair follicle keratinocytes, Langerhans cells, monocytes, macrophages, dermal fibroblasts	• Receptors to ACTH MC2-R are expressed in skin melanocytes, hair follicle cells, keratinocytes, sebaceous and eccrine glands' cells, fibroblasts, muscles, and blood vessels	• Stimulation of cortisol and cortocosterone production • Melanogenesis • Cytokine production • Cell proliferation • Melanocyte dendrite formation • Hair growth • Regulation of immune response and inflammation

Continued on p. 36

Beginning of Table I-1-3 on p. 35

STRESS MEDIATOR	SOURCE	EFFECTOR UNIT	FUNCTIONS
Cortisol	• Adrenal cortex • Skin: hair follicle cells, melanocytes, fibroblasts	• The glucocorticoid receptor is expressed ubiquitously in all skin cells	• Major effects on the immune and inflammatory system • Cell proliferation and survival through the PI3K/Akt pathway • Hair follicle proliferation and differentiation • Epidermal barrier formation
Neurotrophins	• Central nervous system • Neurons of the sympathetic nervous system of the skin • Skin: mast cells, T- and B-cells, keratinocytes, fibroblasts, and melanocytes	• The two receptors, TrK and p75, are expressed in mast cells, immune cells, keratinocytes, fibroblasts, and melanocytes	• Promote skin innervation • Promote mast cell survival and differentiation and modify the expression of inflammatory cytokines • Promote keratinocyte proliferation • Important for the migration, viability, and differentiation of melanocytes and their protection against oxidative stress and apoptosis • Promote differentiation and migration of fibroblasts and possibly the reduction and secretion of matrix metalloproteinases (MMPs)
Prolactin	• Pituitary gland • Skin: hair follicle cells and epidermal keratinocytes, fibroblasts, adipocytes, sweat glands and sebaceous glands	• The prolactin receptor is expressed ubiquitously except in fibroblasts	• Autocrine modulator of hair growth by stimulating catagen (hair regression); • Stimulates keratinocyte growth and keratin production in keratinocytes, as well as sebum production in sebaceous glands • Immunomodulatory agent

Continued on p. 37

STRESS MEDIATOR	SOURCE	EFFECTOR UNIT	FUNCTIONS
Substance P	• Sensory nerve fibers	• Mast cells, macrophages, T-cells	• Induction of inflammation, mast cell activation, lymphocyte proliferation • Increases vascular permeability
Catechol-amines (adrenaline and norepi-nephrine)	• Adrenal me-dulla • Nerve fibers of the skin, keratinocytes	• Adrenergic receptors are expressed by natural killer cells, mono-cytes and T-cells, kerati-nocytes, and melanocytes	• Regulate proliferation, differentiation, and migra-tion of keratinocytes • Promote melanogenesis • Reduce fibroblast migra-tion and collagen secretion • Disrupt wound healing • Suppress IL-12 production in dendritic cells, leading to Th1 inhibition and in-creased Th2 differentiation • Important for lympho-cyte turnover, circulation, proliferation, and cytokine production

1.4.7. The nocebo effect

A **nocebo effect** occurs when negative patient expectations re-garding a treatment cause the treatment to have a more negative effect than otherwise would have. For example, when a patient an-ticipates a side effect of a medication, they can experience that effect even if the "medication" is an inert substance (Wikipedia).

The IFSI working group has also identified the nocebo effect as a potential pathogenetic mechanism underlying skin sensitivity (Mis-ery L. et al., 2020). The nocebo effect is the opposite of the placebo effect. It can be characterized as negative effects of treatment not only because of treatment mechanisms but also because of negative pa-tient expectations. Studies show that expectations can significantly in-fluence the results of therapy and the occurrence of certain adverse symptoms (Evers A.W.M. et al., 2018).

The possibility of a nocebo effect in the pathophysiology of sensitive skin is evidenced by studies concerning increased itching and even increased blister size in response to histamine administration in healthy subjects with very negative expectations of the experiment compared to subjects with no expectations (Stumpf A. et al., 2016).

The nocebo effects in a clinical setting were also investigated by Liccardi G. et al. (2004) whose study participants were outpatients that had previously experienced adverse drug reactions. About 27% of patients who took a placebo as a part of a standard exposure protocol demonstrated nocebo reactions such as pruritus and skin lesions.

1.4.8. The microbiome in sensitive skin

The skin microbiome — the association of microorganisms inhabiting the skin — is essential in maintaining skin health. The main part of the "healthy" microbiome is made up of bacteria from the *Actinobacteria*, *Proteobacteria*, *Firmicutes,* and *Bacteroidetes families*, while the genus *Malassezia* dominates among fungi, as *Demodex* mites live there. While viruses are also present, their role is the least studied (Byrd A.L. et al., 2018). The microbiome composition depends on the state of the skin, including the lipids secreted on its surface (which serve as the main source of nutrition for microorganisms), pH, the amount of water, trace elements, etc.

Whether qualitative and quantitative changes in the microbiome composition are the cause or consequence of various skin diseases remains to be ascertained (in most cases, this is a bilateral process). Still, they have been recorded in many skin pathologies, including acne, atopic dermatitis, psoriasis, and rosacea.

This influence is associated not only with the development of inflammatory rash but also with a direct impact on the skin barrier (Baldwin H.E. et al., 2017). Recent studies show that both the diversity of the microbiome and the relative predominance of some "good" microorganisms over conditionally pathogenic ones play a role in the formation of a healthy barrier. Accordingly, adverse changes in these indicators (impoverishment or shift in proportions), cause a violation of its normal structure and function. Still, many scientists agree that there are no typical microbiomes in certain diseases, as communities can change individually. Paraphrasing the first sentence of Leo Tolstoy's novel *Anna Karenina* — "Happy families are all alike; every unhappy family is unhappy in its way" — scientists have put forward a so-called Anna Karenina hypothesis, which states "Healthy microbiomes are all alike; every unhealthy microbiome is unhealthy in its way" (Ma Z.S., 2020). Moreover, **the more the microbiome composition changes** (deviates from a balanced state), **the more the skin barrier function deteriorates** (Yuan C. et al., 2020).

Of course, the microbiome factor is also implicated in the sensitive skin syndrome. As mentioned above, impaired permeability of the skin barrier is one of the pathogenetic mechanisms of this condition. Therefore, dysbiosis leading to a related problem may increase skin sensitivity. In addition, our innate immune system is responsible for interacting with the microbiome. A key role in innate immunity is played by Toll-like receptors (TLR) and the cathelicidin pathway (Kligman A.M., 2001).

Toll-like receptors type 2 (TLR2) is a class of transmembrane cell receptors, the detecting part of which is located on the surface of epithelial cells (including keratinocytes) and immune system cells (monocytes/macrophages, neutrophils, dendritic cells, and mast cells). When they encounter various microorganisms, receptors are activated, and the immune response is triggered inside the cell. This initiates a chain of reactions with the release of pro-inflammatory cytokines, chemokines, proteases, and pro-angiogenic factors aimed at fighting the foreign pathogen. The central factor in this process is the cathelicidin antimicrobial peptide (CAMP) and its active form, peptide LL-37, whose action is associated with increased inflammation in the skin, vascular dilation, and proliferation through VEGF, increased neutrophil chemotaxis, and dysregulation of the synthesis of extracellular matrix components. TLR2 activation increases the synthesis of cathelicidin as well as trypsin-like serine protease kallikrein 5 (KLK5), the enzyme by which cathelicidin is converted into LL-37 (Tan J., Berg M., 2013; Scheenstra M.R. et al., 2020).

TLR2 are abundant in mast cells, including those whose degranulation results in histamine release (Igawa S., Di Nardo A., 2017). In addition, they are also found on free nerve endings responsible for the perception of pain and itching (Liu T. et al., 2012). When the microbiome is balanced, the immune system does not show aggressive reactions against its "good" neighbors, but when its composition changes, it begins to react. This eventually leads to the development of inflammation, itching, and pain. In some cases, the inflammation may not be particularly pronounced. Still, if people with sensitive skin have hyperreactivity of nerve fibers, the microbiome imbalance may result in unpleasant symptoms of skin hypersensitivity.

Fig. I-1-11 and **I-1-12** illustrate receptors of nerve endings interacting with different microorganisms and demonstrate how an imbalance in the microbiome can lead to pruritus (Kim H.S., Yosipovitch G., 2020).

Only a few studies directly examining the microbiome of sensitive skin have been conducted to date, and some of the obtained findings

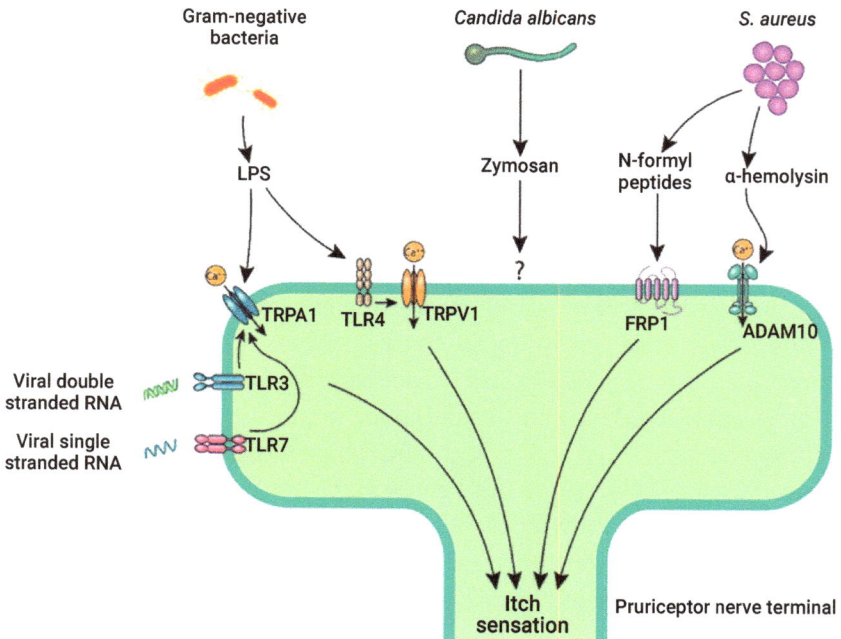

Figure I-1-11. Schematic of the interaction of various potentially pathogenic skin-inhabiting microorganisms with nerve endings (adapted from Kim H.S., Yosipovitch G., 2020)

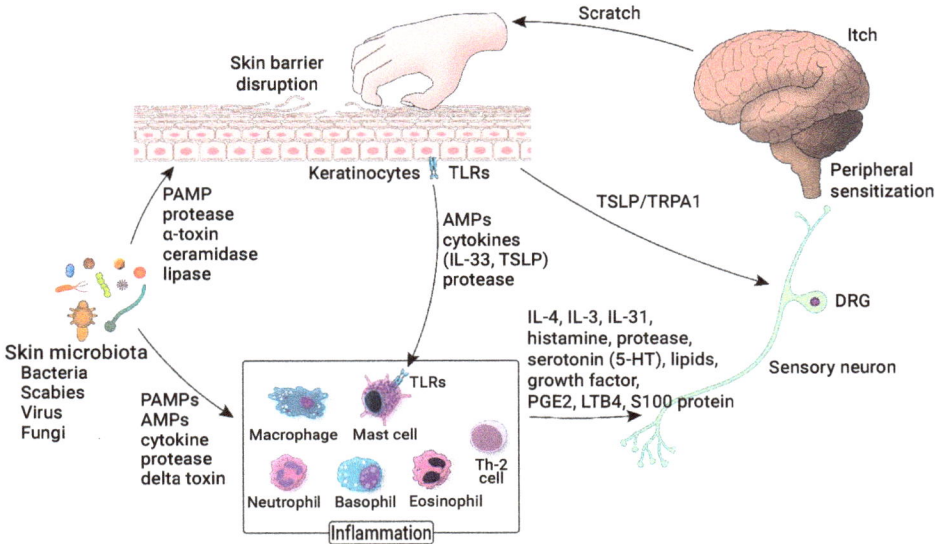

Figure I-1-12. Inflammatory circuit of the skin microbiota. Various microbiota (bacteria, fungi, and viruses) cover the exterior of healthy skin where the barrier is intact. In dysbiosis, pathogens release proteases, which may disrupt the epidermal barrier. Delta-toxin causes mast cell degranulation, which prompts inflammation and itching (adapted from Kim H.S., Yosipovitch G., 2020)

Abbreviations: AMP — antimicrobial peptides; DRG — dorsal root ganglia; IL — interleukin; LTB4: — leukotriene B4; PAMP — pathogen-associated molecular pattern; PGE2 — prostaglandin E2; TLR — Toll-like receptor; TRPA1 — transient receptor potential antigen 1; TSLP — thymic stromal lymphopoietin

suggest no discernible differences in the microbial composition of sensitive and non-sensitive skin (Hillion M. et al., 2013). However, one of the recent works yielded quite interesting results, as Keum H.L. et al. (2020) found that despite the conventionally comparable bacterial composition of sensitive and non-sensitive skin, there are differences in the mycobiome, i.e., in the fungal composition. Along with a decrease in *Malassezia restricta* — the main representative of the genus *Malassezia* on the skin — they also noted an increase in the diversity of other fungi. In addition, they observed a change in the "controlling" interactions between microorganisms.

Another interesting aspect is the relationship between skin sensitivity and the gut microbiome composition. Recent studies point to the role of the gut microbiome in visceral hypersensitivity, anxiety, and depression and support the view that microbial imbalance may contribute to the development and persistence of irritable bowel syndrome (IBS) symptoms (Distrutti E. et al., 2016). In addition, the gut microbiome influences bidirectional communication between the intestinal nervous system and the central nervous system, modulating gut development and several physiological functions, including intestinal peristalsis, sensitivity, secretion, and immunity. Thus, immune system activation and pro-inflammatory cytokine production may indirectly affect the skin. This assertion is supported by a recent study involving 5,000 participants, 13.6% of whom had IBS and 59.1% reported having sensitive skin. As 73.2% of people with IBS also suffered from sensitive skin, the authors concluded that IBS may result in severe skin sensitivity (Seite S., Misery L., 2018).

Part II

Classification and clinical manifestations of sensitive skin syndrome

1.1. Classification of sensitive skin

The pathophysiology of hypersensitivity is still debated in the scientific community without any signs of emerging consensus. This lack of a common position among researchers is also reflected in the diversity of classifications. For example, Japanese dermatologists suggest distinguishing three main types of sensitive skin (Yokota T. et al., 2003):

- **Unprotected type** characterized by reduced barrier function, increased transepidermal water loss (TEWL), and abnormal desquamation.
- **Inflamed type** which tends toward inflammatory changes without a pronounced loss of epidermal barrier function.
- **Neurosensitive type** characterized by the absence of inflammatory symptoms and normal barrier function, suggesting that all problems come from within the body.

More than 20 years ago, Mills and Berger proposed the division of people with hypersensitive skin into the following four groups **according to dermatologic principles** (Mills O.H., Berger R.S., 1991):

- Group 1: patients suffering from chronic dermatologic diseases.
- Group 2: similar to the first, but the clinical manifestation is either minimal or atypical.
- Group 3: healthy individuals with one or more episodes of severe skin trauma (e.g., sunburn or contact allergy) in the past. Even after many years, the injured area is hypersensitive.
- Group 4: all others who do not fall into the above categories. In this group, the phenomena of skin hypersensitivity without prior contact with sensitizers are noted.

A different division into subgroups **according to response to triggers** was put forward by Willis C.M. et al. (2001):

- Group 1: characterized by a pronounced response to any type of external stimuli.
- Group 2: characterized by reaction to a contact material only (rough clothing, cosmetics).
- Group 3: exhibiting a reaction to natural factors only (water, wind, hot/cold temperature).

1.2. Clinical manifestations of the sensitive skin syndrome

What complaints do individuals with sensitive skin typically have? This question is difficult to answer, as in each individual case, the clinical picture is made up of a variety of symptoms that manifest to varying degrees and in varying combinations, as shown in **Table II-1-1**.

Table II-1-1. Symptoms of skin hypersensitivity

SUBJECTIVE FEELINGS (CLAIMED BY THE PATIENT)	VISIBLE SYMPTOMS
• Tightness • Burning • Itching • Tingling • Fever • Warmth • General discomfort	• Redness • Edema • Scaling • Rash

An experienced specialist can deduce from the clinical picture the likely causes of such vivid consequences. However, other conditions need to be ruled out because symptoms of skin hypersensitivity can accompany many other pathologies.

Part III

Diagnosis and differential diagnosis of sensitive skin syndrome

1.1. Diagnosis of hypersensitivity

Unfortunately, there are still no comprehensive and reliable instrumental tests for diagnosing sensitive skin largely due to the wide range of complaints, many of which are difficult to assess objectively. Moreover, it is challenging to determine whether a patient with a low sensitivity threshold is susceptible to just one or a few stimuli.

Therefore, the diagnosis process should start with an interview, focusing on gathering all relevant information, including the patient's complaints. Questions to ask during the consultation include what reactions occur when exposed to what factors, in what conditions, what accompanies them, and how do they develop and resolve. It is also necessary to obtain the patient's life history and clarify the presence of diseases and predisposition to allergic reactions.

For this purpose, the **Skin Sensitivity Scale** developed by a team of scientists led by Dr. Laurent Misery (Misery L. et al., 2014) can be used. When administered, patients rate the following most common manifestations of sensitive skin on a 10-point scale (**Fig. III-1-1**):

1. Skin irritation
2. Tingling
3. Burning
4. Sensations of heat
5. Tautness
6. Itching
7. Pain
8. General discomfort
9. Hot flushes
10. Redness

DEGREE OF OVERALL SKIN IRRITATION DURING THE PAST 3 DAYS

Using a vertical line, indicate the symptoms felt during the past 3 days on the horizontal line (0 = absence of irritation, 10 = intolerable irritation)

⚠ Important: To be completed by the patient.

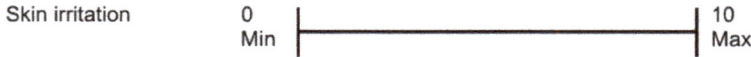

Skin irritation   0 ├─────────────────────────┤ 10
                  Min   Max

SEVERITY OF SKIN CONDITION DURING THE PAST 3 DAYS

Please indicate the intensity of each of the following symptoms during the past 3 days. 0 = zero intensity, 10 = intolerable intensity): darken one number between 0 an 10.

⚠ Important: To be completed by the patient.

Skin condition felt:

	0	1	2	3	4	5	6	7	8	9	10
Tingling	⓪	①	②	③	④	⑤	⑥	⑦	⑧	⑨	⑩
Burning	⓪	①	②	③	④	⑤	⑥	⑦	⑧	⑨	⑩
Sensations of heat	⓪	①	②	③	④	⑤	⑥	⑦	⑧	⑨	⑩
Tautness	⓪	①	②	③	④	⑤	⑥	⑦	⑧	⑨	⑩
Itching	⓪	①	②	③	④	⑤	⑥	⑦	⑧	⑨	⑩
Pain	⓪	①	②	③	④	⑤	⑥	⑦	⑧	⑨	⑩
General discomfort	⓪	①	②	③	④	⑤	⑥	⑦	⑧	⑨	⑩
Hot flashes	⓪	①	②	③	④	⑤	⑥	⑦	⑧	⑨	⑩

Visible skin conditions:

	0	1	2	3	4	5	6	7	8	9	10
Redness	⓪	①	②	③	④	⑤	⑥	⑦	⑧	⑨	⑩

Figure III-1-1. English version of Sensitive Scale-10 (adapted from Misery L. et al., 2014)

The ratings achieved in each domain are summed up to obtain a final score, whereby 20–60 points are indicative of skin sensitivity.

One of the first skin sensitivity tests was proposed by Kligman and Frosch. Their so-called sting test consists of applying lactic acid to the nasolabial folds with subsequent assessment of the intensity of symptoms by the patient (Frosch P.J., Kligman A.M., 1977). However, the test was later shown to be invalid since the patients had varied reactions to the same stimuli. Marriott M. et al. (2005) further established that sensitivity to one substance does not necessarily have to be accompanied by sensitivity to other factors.

Accordingly, this test was substituted by the topical application of capsaicin as this modern test gives accurate results. It was proposed for cutaneous neurosensitivity detection and as a tool for the differential diagnosis of skin hypersensitivity (Green B.G., Shaffer G.S., 1992). Methods such as temperature measurement, tingling test, sodium lauryl sulfate occlusive application, itch assessment, allergy test (Fonacier L., Noor I., 2018), transdermal water loss assessment, corneometry, laser Doppler velocimetry, colorimetry, desquamation measurement, and quantitative sensory test can also be used for diagnosing of sensitive skin (the last method is time-consuming and its use is mostly limited to clinical studies).

As can be seen from **Table III-1-1**, practitioners have various diagnostic tools at their disposal to determine many indicators of skin condition. Although the results will not provide a direct answer, a comprehensive evaluation will help them make the most accurate diagnosis.

Table III-1-1. Parameters considered in the evaluation of sensitive skin

FUNCTIONAL PARAMETER	TEST METHOD
Oiliness	Sebumetry
Moisturization	Corneometry (water in the *stratum corneum*)
Barrier function	Tewametry (TEWL index)
pH	pH-metry
Hyperemia	Evaluation of erythema (hemoglobin content measurement)
Scaling	Wood's lamp examination

1.2. Differential diagnosis

When communicating with a patient, it is important not just to establish sensitive skin syndrome, but also to distinguish it from a skin disease, as well as from neuropsychiatric symptoms (neuroses, hypochondria, dysmorphophobia, distorted body image, chronic fatigue syndrome, etc.). The goal of the differential diagnosis is to identify any differences in sensations from those peculiar to certain dermatoses, as well as compare the duration of reactions and the presence of trigger factors. On the other hand, as sensitive skin syndrome can accompany different skin diseases, this factor must be considered in the prescribed treatment.

Today, experts recommend that, when sensitive skin syndrome is suspected, the following skin pathologies are included in the differential diagnosis, as all are also accompanied by skin hypersensitivity and erythema (Do L.H.D. et al., 2020):

- Atopic dermatitis
- Chemical irritant contact dermatitis
- Phototoxic contact dermatitis (aka photo-irritant contact dermatitis)
- Physical irritant contact dermatitis
- Allergic contact dermatitis
- Photoallergy
- Rosacea

Table III-1-2 summarizes the main features of each disease and how they are diagnosed, with more detailed information below.

Table III-1-2. Conditions associated with skin hypersensitivity and erythema (Do L.H.D. et al., 2020)

PATHOLOGY	MANIFESTATIONS	RECOMMENDED STUDIES
Atopic dermatitis	Erythema, scaling	History, physical examination
Chemical irritant contact dermatitis	Erythema, hyperkeratosis, or blistering cracks in certain areas	Anamnesis, patch test to identify stimuli
Phototoxic contact dermatitis		
Physical irritant contact dermatitis		
Allergic contact dermatitis	Visible erythema at the site of contact	Patch test for allergen detection
Photoallergy	Erythema, blistering in the sun-exposed area of the skin after application of certain products	Life history, medication history (drugs or cosmetics)
Rosacea	Transient or persistent erythema with flare-ups and a feeling of fever	Medical history, in some cases a biopsy may be necessary

1.2.1. Atopic dermatitis

Atopic dermatitis is a chronic inflammatory skin disease in individuals with a hereditary predisposition. The incidence of atopic dermatitis is much higher among children (17–24%) compared to adults (4–7%). The disease manifests itself during the first six months of life in 45% of patients and by the age of five in 85% of cases. Only half of the children suffering from atopic dermatitis have persistent remission in adulthood (Czarnowicki T. et al., 2017).

There are two key factors in the pathogenesis of atopic dermatitis:
- Immune dysregulation
- Impaired skin barrier function

The question of which of them is primary is still open. According to the traditional ideas about the pathogenesis of atopic dermatitis, the first place is occupied by abnormal T-cells, which enter the dermis with the bloodstream and provoke an inflammatory reaction. Inflammation disrupts the homeostasis of the epidermis. As a result, the *stratum corneum* is formed incorrectly and ceases to cope with the barrier function. In other words, damage to the *stratum corneum* results from inflammation (**inside-out scenario**). It thus follows that, if the inflammation is extinguished, the homeostasis of the underlying layers is restored.

In contrast, the **outside-in scenario** suggests that an abnormal *stratum corneum* is the first link in the pathogenetic chain. Foreign agents enter the skin through this weak barrier, and the immune system responds with inflammation. To date, several genetic mutations have been identified, affecting different aspects in the skin barrier maturation. Accordingly, the disease course severity depends on the type of "breakage" (including very severe variants, such as ichthyosis and Netherton's syndrome).

Both scenarios share common mechanisms that lead to chronic inflammation. Each of these mechanisms will be discussed in this book as a potential target for therapeutic intervention.

The diagnostic criteria for atopic dermatitis were first proposed by Hanifin J. and Rajka H. in 1980 and have since been revised to indicate that diagnosing atopic dermatitis requires three major and three minor criteria (**Fig. III-1-2**).

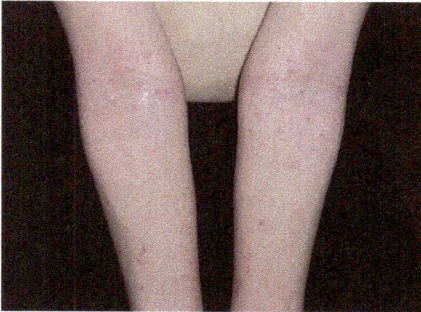

Excoriated papules, lichenification

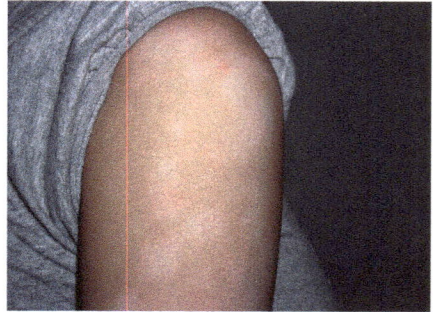

Dyschromia

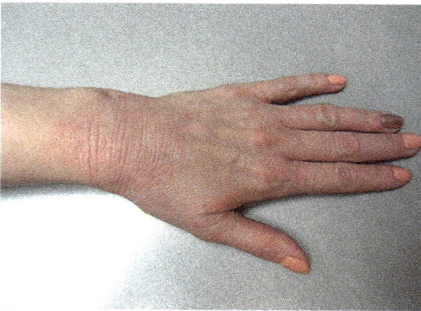

Hand lesions

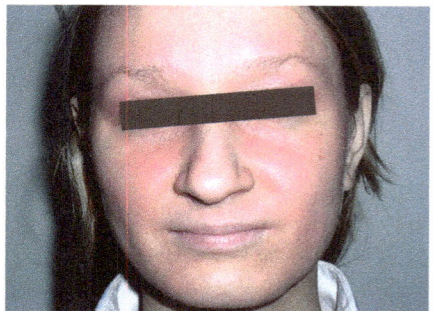

Cosmetics intolerance in a patient with atopic dermatitis

Figure III-1-2. Manifestations of atopic dermatitis (Photo: Albanova V.I.)

Main criteria

- Itching
- Typical clinical picture and localization of rashes
- Chronic recurrent manifestation
- Presence of concomitant atopy (bronchial asthma, allergic rhinitis, conjunctivitis)
- Starts in infancy or early childhood
- Hereditary predisposition and atopy in the family
- Presence of allergen-specific IgE in the history, actual or expected (children in the first year of life) in the peripheral blood and/ or in the skin

Additional (secondary) diagnostic criteria

- Dry skin
- Ichthyosis vulgaris
- Atopic palms (creasing and dryness of the palms, intensification of the skin pattern)
- Follicular keratosis
- Tendency toward allergic dermatitis and eczema on the hands and feet (in adults)
- Persistent white dermographism
- Frequent pyoderma
- Frequent episodes of herpes simplex
- Recurrent conjunctivitis
- Face pallor or erythema
- Periorbital skin darkening
- Rarefaction of the outer part of the eyebrows
- Longitudinal folds of the lower eyelid (Denny–Morgan lines)
- Keratoconus, anterior subcapsular cataract
- Cheilitis
- Geographic tongue
- Folding of the anterior surface of the neck
- The "dirty neck" symptom (dark patches on the neck)
- White lichen
- Secondary leukoderma
- Breast nipple dermatitis
- Drug allergies
- Hives
- Increased itching at night and at sweating
- Provoking influence of emotional, nutritional, climatic, infectious, and other factors
- Seasonality of exacerbations

1.2.2. Chemical irritant contact dermatitis

Chemical irritant contact dermatitis (also known as simple contact dermatitis or simple irritant dermatitis) develops in response to contact with a caustic or toxic substance. Its severity depends on the concentration of the irritant, its chemical structure, the state of the *stratum corneum*, and other factors (Tan C.H. et al., 2014).

For example, the surfactant sodium lauryl sulfate (used in household detergents and shampoos as a detergent and in cheap creams as an emulsifier) causes skin irritation at 0.75% concentration. Due to its high irritant potential, sodium lauryl sulfate is the "gold standard" in model irritation tests. Chemical modification, such as replacing sulfate with phosphate or ethoxylation (conversion to sodium laureth sulfate) and combination with other surfactants (e.g., cocamidopropyl betaine), can reduce the irritant potential of sodium lauryl sulfate. In case of damage, repeated action of irritants, or prolonged hyperhydration of the *stratum corneum*, all irritants begin to act at lower concentrations. Although many substances with the potential to damage skin cells can be found in cosmetic formulations, they are usually present in concentrations that do not cause skin and eye irritation in experimental animals. Nevertheless, for some people, even these low concentrations are sufficient to cause contact dermatitis.

The following ingredients may pose a risk to such individuals (Simion F.A. et al., 1995):

- **Surfactants** included as detergents (in detergents) or emulsifiers (in cosmetic emulsions). Accordingly, people with hypersensitivity and/or damaged barrier (e.g., after peeling or mesotherapy) are advised to use special formulations for skin cleansing, especially those designed for dry skin. Traditional emulsions should also be avoided if possible and should be replaced with lamellar-based products that do not contain surfactants (in this case, manufacturers usually note that the product "does not contain surfactants" or "based on a lamellar structure").

- **Natural soap** as it destroys the *stratum corneum* due to highly active surfactants, and has an alkaline reaction (pH 9–11), which negatively affects the activity of the *stratum corneum* enzymes. Even people with normal skin are not advised to leave the soap solution on the skin for a long time. It is better to soap up a few times and rinse off quickly rather than increase the exposure time.

- **Alcohol and acetone (universal solvents)** as these substances destroy the hydrolipidic film and disrupt the skin barrier integrity, thus allowing foreign substances to enter the skin.
- **Acids** that are used for chemical peels or in pre-peel products.

1.2.3. Phototoxic contact dermatitis

Dose-dependent phototoxic reactions can occur in any person. Due to the interaction of photons with a chemical, a photochemical reaction develops in the skin, resulting in the formation of reactive oxygen species that cause cell damage. The severity of the phototoxic reaction depends on the properties of the chemical, such as skin absorption, metabolism, chemical stability, and solubility. The phototoxic reaction is at the heart of photodynamic therapy (PDT), where absorption of photons by photosensitizer molecules in the presence of oxygen leads to a photochemical reaction that converts molecular triplet oxygen into singlet oxygen and produces many highly reactive radicals causing necrosis and/or apoptosis in target cells (Lee Y.S. et al., 2017; Sun C.Y. et al., 2018).

Phototoxic contact dermatitis occurs after a single skin contact with a chemical without the involvement of immune hypersensitivity reactions. The resulting lesion has a clear border, and after the resolution of inflammation, visible desquamation and/or persistent hyperpigmentation of the affected skin develops.

Phototoxic reactions caused by doxycycline, tetracycline, fluoroquinolones, quinine, furocoumarins, and some other drugs can manifest as nail plate opacity, subungual hyperkeratosis, and onycholysis (Goetze S. et al., 2017; Negulescu M. et al., 2017; Soeur J. et al., 2017).

It is also important to note that some commonly used systemic medications can increase skin sensitivity to UV radiation. We have listed the most common photosensitizers with a high risk of phototoxic (associated with direct cellular damage and accelerating sunburn) and photoallergic (immune dermatitis-like events) reactions in **Table III-1-3**. Therefore, when gathering patient's medical history, the use of these drugs (and even perfume use) must be documented.

Table III-1-3. Photosensitizers

DRUGS	PHOTOTOXIC REACTION	PHOTOALLERGIC REACTION
Antibiotics		
Tetracyclines (doxycycline, tetracycline)	Yes	No
Fluoroquinolones (ciprofloxacin, ofloxacin, levofloxacin)	Yes	No
Sulfonamides	Yes	No
Antiviral drugs		
Acyclovir	No	Yes
Non-steroidal anti-inflammatory drugs		
Ibuprofen	Yes	No
Ketoprofen	Yes	Yes
Naproxen	Yes	No
Celecoxib	No	Yes
Hormonal drugs		
Hydrocortisone	No	Yes
Diuretics		
Furosemide	Yes	No
Bumetanide	No	No
Hydrochlorothiazide	Yes	No
Retinoids		
Isotretinoin	Yes	No
Acitretin	Yes	No
Hypoglycemic drugs		
Sulfonylureas (glipizide, glyburide)	No	Yes
HMG-CoA reductase inhibitors		
Statins (atorvastatin, fluvastatin, lovastatin, pravastatin, simvastatin)	Yes	Yes
Epidermal growth factor inhibitors		
Cetuximab, panitumumab, erlotinib, gefitinib, lapatinib, vandetanib	Yes	Yes

Continued on p. 57

DRUGS	PHOTOTOXIC REACTION	PHOTOALLERGIC REACTION
Antipsychotic drugs		
Phenothiazines (chlorpromazine, fluphenazine, fluphenazine, perazine, perphenazine, thioridazine)	Yes	Yes
Thioxanthenes (chlorprothixene, thiothixene)	Yes	No
Antifungal drugs		
Terbinafine	No	No
Itraconazole	Yes	Yes
Voriconazole	Yes	No
Griseofulvin	Yes	Yes
Other drugs		
5-Fluorouracil	Yes	Yes
Paclitaxel	Yes	No
Amiodarone	Yes	No
Diltiazem	Yes	No
Quinidine	Yes	Yes
Hydroxychloroquine	No	No
Nifedipine	Yes	No
Enalapril	No	No
Dapsone	No	Yes
Oral contraceptives	No	Yes
Alpha-hydroxy acids		
Glycolic acid	Yes (in high concentration)	Yes
Sunscreens		
Para-aminobenzoic acid	No	Yes
Cinnamic acid esters (cinnamates)	No	Yes
Benzophenones	No	Yes
Salicylates	No	Yes

Continued on p. 58

DRUGS	PHOTOTOXIC REACTION	PHOTOALLERGIC REACTION
Flavorings		
Amber musk	No	Yes
6-Methylcoumarin	No	Yes
Essential oils (bergamot, cumin, ginger, lemon, lime, tangerine, orange, and verbena)	No (with the exception of bergamot)	Yes

1.2.4. Physical irritant contact dermatitis

A variety of factors of a physical nature can trigger neurogenic inflammation, including:

- Low and high temperature (thermal urticaria)
- Sunlight
- Friction
- Prolonged squeezing
- Vibration

1.2.5. Allergic contact dermatitis

A distinctive feature of allergic dermatitis is that the severity of skin irritation does not depend on the concentration of the allergen. In allergy, immune cells first **memorize** a substance (allergen) and **sensitize** (i.e., increase the body's sensitivity to the allergen). When the skin comes into contact with the substance next time, an immune reaction accompanied by inflammation develops. Once the immune cells register the presence of the substance, they develop a large-scale inflammatory reaction. In most cases, this reaction remains local and is characterized by blisters and erythema (e.g., allergic urticaria), but in rare instances, the allergic reaction can develop into a potentially fatal complication — anaphylaxis accompanied by pulmonary edema.

According to the data published in popular press sources, allergic contact dermatitis accounts for almost 70% of all reactions to cosmetics. However, it is almost impossible to say how close to reality this figure is given that consumers usually call any negative reaction "allergy" (although in medicine, specific immune processes are associated with this condition). Moreover, most consumers who encounter skin irritation do not consult doctors (and therefore do not get included in such estimates) and either simply change the brand of cosmetics or refuse to use them. Therefore, most experts believe that allergic reactions comprise a small percentage of all reactions to cosmetics. Nevertheless, they are the most studied (Jack A.R. et al., 2013; Park M.E., Zippin J.H., 2014).

Although any substance in a cosmetic product can be an allergen for a particular person, cosmetic ingredients differ in allergenicity. According to the frequency with which allergies to this component occur, allergenicity can be low, medium, or high. The last category includes preservatives, especially those that release formaldehyde, some UV filters, and fragrances, both natural (essential oils) and synthetic (**Tables III-1-4** and **III-1-5**). Still, not all these substances are true allergens, as some (e.g., oxybenzone) increase skin sensitivity to sunlight and are photosensitizers.

Table III-1-4. Some components of cosmetic products causing skin sensitization (according to the current European Cosmetics Directive, EU Cosmetics Directive 76/768/EEC)

INCI	CHEMICAL NATURE	COMMENTS
2-Bromo-2-nitro-propane-1,3-diol DMDM hydantoin Imidazolidinyl urea Diazolidinyl urea Quaternium-15	Substances releasing formaldehyde	Preservatives
Methylparaben Propylparaben	Parabens: methyl-4-hydroxy-benzoate and propyl-4-hy-droxybenzoate	Preservatives
Methylchloroiso-thiazolinone (and) methylisothiazo-linone	A mixture of two preservatives	A preservative acceptable for use in products that need to be rinsed off, such as shampoos
Parfume	Fragrances (synthetic and in essential oils)	Giving the product a pleasant odor

Continued on p. 60

INCI	CHEMICAL NATURE	COMMENTS
Lanolin and its derivatives	Lanolin (wool wax, animal wax) is a mixture of esters of high molecular weight alcohols (cholesterol, isocholesterol, etc.) with fatty containing 6 and more carbons (myristic, palmitic, cerotic, etc.) and free high-molecular-weight alcohols.	Emollient
Colophonium	Rosin is a solid constituent of resinous substances of coniferous trees, remaining after distillation of volatile substances. It contains 60–92% of resin acids (mainly abietic acid), 0.5–12% of saturated and unsaturated fatty acids, and 8–20% of neutral substances (sesqui-, di- and triterpenoids).	In the cosmetics industry, pine rosin of grade a (1st grade) is used in lipsticks, manicure varnishes and varnish-pastes at a concentration of up to 4.0%.
Tosylamide/form-aldehyde resin	Tosylamide/formaldehyde resin	Included in the base of nail polish, releases formaldehyde
p-Phenylenedi-amine p-Toluenediamine	para-Phenylenediamine para-Toluenediamine	Hair dyes
Butylhydroxytolu-ene (BHT)	Butylhydroxytoluene Ionol	Lipophilic antioxidant, synthetic analog of vitamin E, also used as a food preservative
Benzophenone-3	Oxybenzone	UVA/B filter, in concentrations more 0.5% may increase skin sensitivity to sunlight (photosensitization)
Butyl me-thoxydibenzoyl-methane	Avobenzone	Oil-soluble UVA filter that rapidly degrades in the light, therefore it is necessary to stabilize it (e.g., with oxocrylene, cyclodextrins, etc.)
Octyl dimethyl-para-aminoben-zoic acid (octyl dimethyl-PABA)	PABA derivative	UVB filter, may cause contact dermatitis or increase skin sensitivity to sunlight (photo-sensitization)

Continued on p. 61

INCI	CHEMICAL NATURE	COMMENTS
Ethylhexyl methoxycinnamate	Cinnamic acid derivative	UVB filter, oil-soluble, max. permissible concentration 7.5%
Resorcinol	Dihydroxybenzene resorcinol	It is used as an antiseptic and disinfectant agent at 5–10% in oily phase in anti-dandruff shampoos, and in Jessner peel solution

Table III-1-5. Substances (International Nomenclature of Cosmetic Ingredients, INCI) used as fragrances that must be separately listed in the ingredients list if their concentration exceeds 0.001% in leave-on products and 0.01% in rinse-off products (according to the current European Cosmetics Directive, EU Cosmetics Directive 76/768/EEC)

- alpha-Isomethyl ionone
- Amyl cinnamal
- Amylcinnamyl alcohol
- Anise alcohol
- Benzyl alcohol
- Benzyl benzoate
- Benzyl cinnamate
- Benzyl salicylate
- Butylphenyl methylpropional
- Cinnamal
- Cinnamyl alcohol
- Citral
- Citronellol
- Coumarin
- Eugenol
- *Evernia prunastri, Evernia furfuracea*
- Farnesol
- Geraniol
- Hexyl cinnamal
- Hydroxycitronellal
- Hydroxyisohexyl 3-cyclohexene carboxaldehyde
- Isoeugenol
- Limonene
- Linalool
- Methyl 2-octynoate

Fragrances are the most dangerous allergens, yet they are anonymized in most cosmetics in the list of ingredients and are simply denoted as *Parfum* or *Fragrance*. From a dermatological point of view, this is incorrect since fragrances differ in their chemical nature and degree of danger they pose to the skin. **Table III-1-5** shows the 25 fragrances identified as the most allergenic, which by law must be listed separately from the word *Parfum* if their concentration exceeds 0.001% in leave-on products and 0.01% in rinse-off products (e.g., shampoos or cleansing milk).

As those with food allergies to nuts should avoid cosmetics containing nut extracts, **Table III-1-6** lists the most commonly occurring nuts with their Latin name (also used in the International Nomenclature of Cosmetic Ingredients, INCI) and their common name in English. To determine the allergenicity of a particular ingredient, a repeated patch test is used, whereby occlusive patches with the substance are first applied to 50–200 volunteers, and then, after some time, the application is repeated, but on a different area of the skin.

Table III-1-6. Nut "sources" of cosmetic ingredients

LATIN NAME / INCI	COMMON NAME
Prunus amygdalus *Prunus amara*	Almond Bitter almond
Prunus dulcis	Sweet almond
Bertholletia excelsa	Brazil nut
Anacardium occidentale	Cashew nut
Castanea sativa	Chestnut
*Cocos nucifera**	Coconut*
Corylus avellana *Corylus americana* *Corylus rostrata*	Hazelnut
Aesculus hippocastanum	Horse chestnut
Cola vera	Kola nut
Aleurites muluccana	Kukui nut
Macadamia ternifolia *Macadamia integrifolia*	Macadamia nut
Arachis hypogaea	Peanut
Pistacia vera *Pistacia lentiscus*	Pistachio nut
Juglans regia *Juglans mandshurica* *Juglans nigra*	Walnut
Sesamum indicum	Sesame seed

* In rare cases, coconut causes food allergy.

1.2.6. Photoallergy

Photoallergic reaction occurs in sensitized individuals when a photosensitizing drug or chemical substance repeatedly interacts with solar or UV radiation. Photoallergy occurs about half an hour after the onset of UV exposure and then spreads to areas of the skin that are shielded from exposure. In photoallergic reactions, unlike phototoxic reactions, the lesion boundaries are less clearly demarcated, and their resolution is not accompanied by skin hyperpigmentation.

Drugs, chemicals, or their metabolites, while absorbing photons, form photoactive compounds in the skin, which acquire immunogenic properties and initiate cell-mediated immune reactions of delayed-type hypersensitivity. Photoallergy is often caused by cosmetics and perfumes containing musk, ambergris, orange, bergamot, and lemon essential oils, sandalwood oil, as well as some drugs, such as ibuprofen (Khandpur S. et al., 2017; Onoue S. et al., 2017).

1.2.7. Rosacea

Rosacea occupies a special place in the differential diagnosis of sensitive skin, as these two conditions are often considered side by side in clinical practice, as well as in some scientific publications. Indeed, they have quite a lot in common, but they are separate conditions. As rosacea is discussed in detail in our book *Rosacea and Couperosis in the Cosmetic Dermatology & Skincare Practice*, in this section, we will only briefly summarize the main points important for diagnosing this disease.

Rosacea is a chronic, recurrent facial skin disease based on angioneurotic disorders. It is polyetiological and is characterized by a staged manifestation.

Many factors are involved in the pathogenesis of rosacea, as well as in the pathogenesis of sensitive skin, including TLR2 receptors, TRP channels, mast cells, skin barrier structures, skin and microbiome. It is currently believed that rosacea is caused by a combination of immune system disorders, changes in vascular reactivity, and abnormalities in the perception and transmission of nerve signals, deterioration of the skin barrier function, and microbiome dysbiosis underpinned by genetic predisposition, which ultimately leads to increased skin sensitivity and inflammation. It is important to note that a combination of factors is usually implicated, and in many cases, the involved processes interact.

Currently, there are two main classifications of rosacea. The first, which has already become classic, was proposed back in 2002 and is based on the allocation of four rosacea subtypes according to clinical symptoms (Wilkin J. et al., 2002):

1. Erythematouteleangiectatic (centrofacial)
2. Papulopustular (inflammatory, acneiform)
3. Phymatous
4. Ocular (ophthalmic rosacea)

In addition, special forms of rosacea have been identified (Wilkin J. et al., 2002):

- Granulomatous
- Steroidal
- Gram-negative
- Conglobate
- Fulminant

Four distinct **stages of rosacea** are also recognized:

- **Stage 1 — Pre-Rosacea:** At this initial stage, the facial redness flashes are transient and disappear soon after the cause or trigger is removed. Moreover, a functional change can occur whereby the blood vessels start to dilate in response to more stimuli than before, they start to open wider than before, and begin to stay open for longer periods. There are no physical signs of vascular damage.
- **Stage 2 — Mild Rosacea:** This stage begins when the facial redness continues for a long time (half an hour or more) because facial blood vessels remain open even after the trigger has been removed. The skin is often described as rosy or as having a healthy-looking glow. Minor structural damage may be visible.
- **Stage 3 — Moderate Rosacea:** This stage begins when the facial redness persists for days or even weeks, as facial blood vessels can show different levels of structural damage. In some cases, there is a semi-permanent redness in the central area covering the nose and cheeks. The face is often described as having

a sun-burned or wind-burned look. In most cases, there are prominent areas of telangiectasia where flashing is more pronounced. Some sufferers also report swelling and/or burning sensations, as well as outbreaks of inflammatory papules and pustules. The papules result from inflammatory substances escaping from damaged vessels and migrating to the superficial layers of the skin.

- **Stage 4 — Severe Rosacea:** This stage is a result of uncontrolled facial flashing over an extended period. Although a few moderate rosacea sufferers progress to this most severe form, it is characterized by intense episodes of facial flashing, severe inflammation, swelling, and debilitating burning sensations. This inflammation is typically accompanied by crops of inflammatory papules, pustules, and nodules, and some people develop phymatous changes in certain areas of the face. The major changes that have occurred by this stage include widespread damage to the facial blood vessels, extreme hyperreactivity of the remaining blood vessels, significant leakage from damaged blood vessel walls, and adverse changes to the facial skin structure.

Persistent erythema in the central part of the face that has persisted for three months is considered a mandatory clinical sign of rosacea, while optional attributes indicating the stages of the disease include:

1. Telangiectasias
2. Papules
3. Pustules
4. Phymatous skin changes

This classification has helped systematize the symptoms of rosacea, allowing clinicians to review the most appropriate approaches to therapy at each stage. However, despite its widespread use, it has shortcomings, as it ignores other symptoms of rosacea not described by clinical forms and does not consider the overlap among subtypes. Moreover, new information about the pathogenesis of rosacea has emerged over the years, changing our understanding of the disease.

Therefore, in 2017, the expert committee of the US National Rosacea Society proposed an updated classification that emphasized a more patient-centered phenotypic approach shown in **Table III-1-7** (Gallo R.L. et al., 2018). According to this most recent classification, at least one diagnostic feature or two primary features are sufficient to diagnose rosacea, whereas secondary signs (irrespective of their number) are not considered a diagnostic criterion but rather serve as a complement for the main signs. The specific treatment type and approach to the therapy, as well as the severity of the disease, will depend on the combination of signs from all three main groups.

Table III-1-7. New 2017 classification of rosacea by the US National Rosacea Society based on the diagnostic, primary, and secondary features of rosacea (Gallo R.L. et al., 2018)

DIAGNOSTIC SIGNS	KEY FEATURES	SECONDARY ATTRIBUTES

• Persistent centrofacial erythema aggravated by triggering factors
• Phymatous changes
	• Hot flushes/transient erythema
	• Inflammatory papules and pustules
	• Telangiectasias
	• Ocular manifestations:
	  – telangiectasias along the eyelid margin
	  – conjunctival injection (redness and dilation of blood vessels at the vaults of the conjunctiva, i.e., around the perimeter of the eyeball)
	  – blepharitis, keratitis, conjunctivitis, and sclerokeratitis
		• Burning
		• Tingling
		• Edema
		• Feeling of dryness

It is also important to note that, while rosacea almost always leads to the emergence of sensitive skin symptoms, the reverse is not the case. Thus, skin hypersensitivity alone is not enough to diagnose rosacea.

Part IV

Sensitive skin care

Patients with sensitive skin syndrome may become a real "headache" for skincare practitioners as their unpleasant symptoms are typically caused by cosmetic products. That is why some practitioners are overly cautious, preferring an approach close to "non-intervention" based on excluding many necessary care products from use to determine their impact on the patient's condition. However, a differentiated approach based on the knowledge of the provoking factors, basic mechanisms of skin hypersensitivity, and considering the peculiarities of a particular patient is more effective, as it helps in formulating an individualized treatment protocol aimed at improving the skin condition, as well as the quality of life of the patient.

Although not everything can be cured, the encouraging fact is that most conditions associated with skin hypersensitivity are acquired rather than genetic. Even in special cases, such as atopic dermatitis, much can be done based on pathophysiology. Thus, a gentle approach is always advised when working with sensitive skin, which requires less aggressive exposure, fewer components, reasonable use of procedures, moderate temperatures, and gentle touch (Draelos Z.D., 2000, 2002; Simion F.A., Rau A.H., 2002).

Thus far, we have examined in detail at the pathophysiologic mechanisms of sensitive skin syndrome to understand what types of care would be helpful. The following areas will be discussed next:

- Limiting triggering factors and skin protection
- Gentle cleansing
- Restoring and strengthening the barrier function
- Moisturizing
- Decreasing the excitability of the skin receptors
- Reducing inflammation (including neurogenic inflammation)

This comprehensive approach can significantly alleviate the condition of sensitive skin, and thus improve the patient's quality of life and provide an opportunity for other aesthetic interventions.

Chapter 1
Cosmetic care for sensitive skin

1.1. Limiting triggering factors

The first step is to eliminate (if possible) or limit exposure to the triggers. The patients should avoid the following physical aggressors, mechanical damage, chemical substances, and cosmetic products.

Physical aggressors
- Reduce exposure to direct sunlight and wind
- Use safe sunscreen
- Avoid excessively high or low temperature
- Use humidifiers during the heating season

Mechanical damage
- Do not use loofahs, rough towels, scrubs, and other products that can damage the *stratum corneum*.
- Replace microdermabrasion and brushing with other, gentler cleansing options, such as gas-liquid or ultrasonic peels (if your skin tolerates them normally).
- Avoid aesthetic procedures associated with active mechanical damage to the skin barrier (biorevitalization, mesotherapy, laser resurfacing).
- Intense massage can also worsen the condition and aggravate unwanted symptoms. Gentle and relaxing massages are generally not contraindicated.

Chemical substances
- Don't wash your face with tap water
- Use micellar or thermal water

- Avoid contact with toxic agents (detergents containing aggressive surfactants, detergents, etc.)

Cosmetic products

Cosmetic products containing irritants are not recommended, including:

- Surfactants
- Natural soap
- Alcohol
- Acetone
- Preservatives
- Perfumes
- Alpha-hydroxy acids (AHA) and retinol derivatives in peel products

However, AHA are an exception to the rules outlined above, as if we are dealing with the neurogenic type of hypersensitivity, it is possible to perform peels with a gradual increase in the acid concentration. This is due to the possibility of habituation and desensitization of sensitive fibers. Nonetheless, in all cases, it is necessary to use an individualized approach and monitor the patient's reaction to the procedure, as an undesirable outcome in the form of a pronounced inflammatory reaction is also possible.

The main advice from the IFSI experts is to **limit the use of cosmetics or use products containing little or no preservatives, surfactants, and fragrances even when well-tolerated**. In general, it is advisable to favor cosmetic products with a limited number of ingredients, as the likelihood of triggers among them will also be reduced.

The American Academy of Dermatology recommends following the rules presented below when choosing care and decorative cosmetics to avoid negative side-effects and irritation:

1. **Ensure that the ingredient list is free of potential irritants and toxic agents.** For example, in a study conducted by the US National Rosacea Society, many patients identified the following substances as irritation triggers:
   - Alcohol (66%)
   - Witch hazel extract (30%)

- Fragrances (30%)
- Menthol (21%)
- Mint (14%)
- Eucalyptus essential oil (13%)

Most participants also stated that they avoided tightening agents, exfoliatiants, and other substances potentially harmful to sensitive skin.

2. **Choose products free of fragrances (synthetic fragrances or natural essential oils).** According to the American Academy of Dermatology, "fragrances are more likely to cause contact dermatitis than other substances." Skin is a huge target for exogenous allergens, which can weaken the already weak barrier of sensitive skin. Accordingly, their use increases the risk of irritation. Please note that the label "allergy tested" should not be confused with the label "hypoallergenic" which is not strictly defined in cosmetic legislation.

3. **New products should be tested first.** Before applying a new product to your face, you should test it on another part of your body, such as your neck. If there is an unwanted reaction, don't use it. It is also necessary to carefully read the list of ingredients. The substances that trigger sensitivity symptoms differ from person to person, so it is important to make an individualized list of "forbidden" substances.

4. **If possible, minimize the number of cosmetics used.** It is desirable to choose multifunctional products, as this will reduce their total number. The fewer ingredients they contain, the better.

In addition, a person with sensitive skin should be encouraged to adopt a healthier lifestyle. This can start with those factors that are within personal control and are obvious places for correction, such as avoiding smoking, alcohol and hot drinks, spices, and foods known to cause skin discomfort. Moderate physical activity, as well as practicing yoga and meditation (especially in cases of nervous system lability) is also recommended, as is partaking in alternative hobbies that induce endorphin generation. As we know, endorphins are not only "pleasure hormones" but also have anti-inflammatory properties.

1.2. Protecting sensitive skin

Sun and environmental pollutants are as common triggers of skin sensitivity symptoms as cosmetics. As they also contribute to damage to the skin barrier, individuals with sensitive skin are advised to use skin protective products. However, there are nuances here because, for example, many chemical sunscreens can irritate even the healthy skin as they degrade in the sun and can form potentially toxic compounds.

The 1st generation UV filters such as benzophenone-3 (aka oxybenzone), benzophenone-4, para-aminobenzoic acid (PABA), butyl methoxydibenzoylmethane (Avobenzone), and octocrylene, which have irritant potential and other potentially adverse effects, should be avoided by most individuals, especially those with sensitive skin (Diffey B., 2020). Newer filters like bis-ethylhexyloxyphenol methoxyphenyl triazine (Tinosorb S) have undergone much more research before entering the market and are thus considered more stable and much safer. Moreover, they protect against a wide range of radiation.

In general, physical UV filters such as titanium dioxide and zinc oxide are preferred, as these microparticles reflect radiation in the UVA and UVB spectral range without undergoing chemical transformations. In addition, the irritating potential of physical UV filters is lower than that of chemical filters, which act by absorbing UV rays. However, unlike microparticles, the nanoparticles comprising physical filters have been shown to penetrate the *stratum corneum*, and can leave a whitish film on the skin and even initiate oxidation reactions (Young A.R. et al., 2017).

UV filters based on cerium (Ce) phosphates and oxide/dioxide particles have also been developed. A comparison of the photoprotective properties of cerium oxide with titanium dioxide and zinc dioxide shows an even more pronounced filter efficacy. However, despite the initial hopes of non-toxicity, cerium oxide nanoforms, like other physical filters, are also characterized by potential cytotoxicity and pro-oxidant activity (Miri A. et al., 2020). Thus, micronized forms of all these filters, "packed" in a special shell, are currently considered the safest.

Those with sensitive skin are advised to use sunscreen with a UV index of two or higher. As the UV index (which characterizes the sunlight intensity) is broadcast by many information resources, it is always possible to choose individual sun protection based on the anticipated exposure. For the product to provide the declared photoprotection (sun protection factor [SPF] index), it should be applied at 2 mg/cm² rate and renewed every 2 h (or earlier if the skin was exposed to water in the interim). However, most consumers use about 0.5 mg/cm², rendering sun protection at least four times weaker. All this suggests that SPF is not a guarantee but only a reference point for choosing a product, while noting that the best sunscreen is clothing, hat, and shade.

Sunscreen formulations include substances that impart additional properties to the finished product, such as moisturizing components, anti-inflammatory agents, antioxidants (usually fat-soluble vitamin E), and even immunomodulators (yeast polysaccharides, chitosan), but should still be applied in moderation. As a rule, the higher the degree of photoprotection, the smaller the share of additional "active" components. There is a valid explanation for this relationship: a sunscreen product with a high SPF restrains the "pressure" of UV rays for hours, which means that everything that can potentially increase skin photosensitivity must be avoided. Fragrances and dyes are also highly undesirable, especially for sensitive skin.

Another nuance pertains to the anti-inflammatory agents in sunscreens. Since the only sign of pronounced photodamage to the skin is the appearance of erythema, and anti-inflammatory agents "take it away," there are concerns that their addition to the formula may give people a sense of false security.

On the other hand, the use of photostable antioxidants in the formula is highly recommended, given that they do not reduce the sun protection ability of the product and strengthen the skin's defense against UV free radicals. Moreover, vitamin E directly protects cells from forming cyclobutane pyrimidine dimers in deoxyribonucleic acid (DNA) (Delinasios G.J. et al., 2018).

Ideally, sun exposure between 10 am and 4 pm should be avoided, as this is the period when the sun is at its peak. It should also be remembered that UV exposure increases in the mountains due to the presence of reflective surfaces (snow, water, etc.). Once again, the best sun protection is clothing, hat, and shade.

Products used should also offer protection against environmental pollutants, such as particulate matter (PM), organic compounds, nitrogen, sulfur oxides, etc. Environmental pollution is a huge urban problem, and some experts believe that it also contributes to the sensitive skin epidemic. As extant research shows that most pollutants act by triggering oxidative stress and inflammation (Parrado C. et al., 2019), antioxidant and anti-inflammatory agents are currently considered the main anti-pollution agents.

1.3. Cleansing sensitive skin

Gentle cleansing is perhaps one of the most "vulnerable" steps of caring for sensitive skin, as many triggers of this condition are found in cleansing products.

Still, not washing your skin to avoid the symptoms of skin sensitivity is not an option. The face should be cleaned at least twice a day to remove excess sebum, impurities, microorganisms, as well as cosmetic residues, while avoiding scrubs, sponges, or other mechanical tools that can traumatize the skin. In other words, it is necessary to choose the right cleansers with minimal irritating potential.

1.3.1. Factors determining the irritant potential of a cleanser

pH range

The main irritant factor of a cleanser is the pH. Thanks to the active advertising of cosmetics with a pH of 5.5, many consumers have already memorized that this is the pH of the skin surface. However, recent studies show that the actual pH value is even lower depending on the skin area, and normal pH on the face can be as low as 4.5.

First, what is pH? It is a convenient measure of acidity, calculated as the inverse decimal logarithm of the concentration of hydrogen ions (protons) in a solution. The higher the proton concentration, the greater the acidity. But since the logarithm is inverse, the "numbers" are the opposite: the lower the pH value, the higher the acidity. As neutral solutions have the pH value of 7.0, the pH of acidic solutions is below, and that of alkaline ones is above this value.

The cells of the human body (including skin cells) live in a slightly alkaline environment with the pH 7.1–7.4. Extracellular fluid, intracellular cytoplasm, and blood plasma have normal pH values within slightly alkaline values. However, the skin surface is covered with a layer of dead cells that protect it, like a lizard is protected by its scales. It is only here, in the *stratum corneum*, where there are no living cells, that the pH value is below neutral. The acidic pH on the skin surface is created and maintained by special ingredients of the hydrolipid mantle (Chan A., Mauro T., 2011):

1. Substances secreted to the skin surface as sebum and sweat, such as lactic and butyric acids from sweat, cholesterol sulfate, and free fatty acids (FFA) from sebum. FFA are converted from phospholipids by secretory phospholipase A2*.
2. Metabolic products of natural moisturizing factor (NMF) components such as sodium pyroglutamate and urea.
3. Substances released by microorganisms living on the skin, e.g., *Lactobacillus* bacteria produce lactic acid.
4. Protons generated by Na^+/H^+ antiporters (sodium–hydrogen exchanger-1, NHE1).
5. Carbon dioxide, some amount of which directly escapes from the epidermis and dissolves in the hydrolipid mantle to form carbon dioxide.

In recent years, academic interest in the hydrolipid mantle has grown substantially, as it has become clearer why it is so important to skin health. Studies have shown that the pH gradient through the *stratum corneum* (pH 4.5–5.5 at the surface and 7.0 at the border with the granular layer) regulates keratinization and desquamation. The point is that different enzymes work at different depths of the *stratum corneum*. The surface proteases break down corneodesmosomes (protein "bridges" that bind horny scales to each other), and this is necessary for the scales to exfoliate in time. In deeper layers of the *stratum corneum*, extracellular lipid structures are formed, and other enzymes work in this area. The peculiarity of any enzyme is pH sensitivity; for each enzyme, there is a specific pH range at which it is most active. For instance, for enzymes that regulate desquamation

---

* Phospolipase A2 has been shown to play a central role in the formation of the "acid mantle" in the early maturation of the epidermis postnatally.

near the surface of the *stratum corneum*, the optimal pH value is close to 5.0. For more deeply located enzymes, the optimum shifts to the alkaline direction and becomes about 6.0–7.0. Thus, the **pH gradient is a kind of "switch" that strictly controls the activity of enzymes at different depths of the *stratum corneum***. If the physiological pH gradient is impaired, a failure in the well-balanced mechanisms of maturation and desquamation will occur, leading to a violation of the *stratum corneum* structure. This happens due to exposure of the skin to acidic preparations (based on fruit acids) or washing with alkaline soap. In such cases, the work of enzymes is disturbed and, after some time, visible scaling and increasing dryness of the skin will emerge. If the damaged skin is irrigated with a solution of neutral pH, the restoration of the barrier will be slowed down. Conversely, with a slightly acidic solution, barrier repair will be faster.

In sensitive skin, where not only a barrier but also increased sensory reactivity is involved, both acidic and alkaline environments can activate TRP channels and free nerve endings, causing itching, burning, and other symptoms.

The hydrolipid mantle regulates the microbial community of our skin. A pH of 4.5–5.5 is of evolutionary importance, as it supports a healthy microbiome. In alkalinization, the microbiological balance is disrupted, immediately affecting the skin condition. Specifically, in persons that suffer from acne, a surface pH is about 6.0, which favors excessive growth of *Cutibacterium acnes*. In atopic dermatitis, the surface pH is often elevated, and the microbiome is different from the healthy. When the pH is elevated, a favorable environment for developing purulent bacteria and fungi is created.

Experiments have shown that the surface pH is most noticeably affected by washing and applying cosmetics. After washing with tap water, it takes the skin an average of four hours to regain its pH. If soap is used in washing, this time increases. The use of cosmetic products with a pH greater than 6.0 or less than 4.0 also shifts the pH gradient in the *stratum corneum*, sometimes on purpose.

The question of whether it is advisable to influence the skin by changing the pH gradient in the *stratum corneum* is resolved at other stages of cosmetic care. This is not the task of cleansers, so their pH should not affect the surface pH.

Surfactants

Even if the pH of the cleanser is within the physiological range, the product may still not be 100% safe because surfactants are the main functional ingredients in most formulations, given that the cleanser will not work without them. Surfactants are a mandatory component of cleansers due to their ability to dissolve (emulsify) fats. Still, since both the membranes of living cells and the lipid ctructures of the epidermal barrier contain lipids, we can surmise that **all products that clean the skin well have the potential to damage the epidermal barrier and cell membranes**.

Surfactants are compounds with **amphiphilic structure**, i.e., their molecules have a polar "head" (hydrophilic component: functional groups –OH, –COOH, –O–, etc.) and a non-polar tail (hydrophobic/lipophilic component: hydrocarbon chain). In an aqueous environment, the lipophilic "tail" is embedded in sebum and hydrophobic residues on the skin surface. On the other hand, the hydrophilic "head" faces the water so that the insoluble contamination masses are detached from the skin surface, passed into solution, and washed off (**Fig. IV-1-1**).

Surfactants differ in molecular length, charge, and strength of emulsifying action. The "strongest" surfactants are detergents with high foaming action. Even if the skin is characterized by increased sebum production, prolonged contact with surfactants should be avoided, as its barrier structures and acid mantle may be impaired otherwise.

As surfactant-based cleansers can only work in combination with water, it is no exaggeration to say that **water is the main activator of the cleanser**.

Some surfactants decompose into ions in aqueous solution: anionic surfactants carry a negative charge, cationic surfactants carry a positive charge, and amphoteric surfactants carry both charges. Other surfactants dissolve in water without ionizing (these are so-called

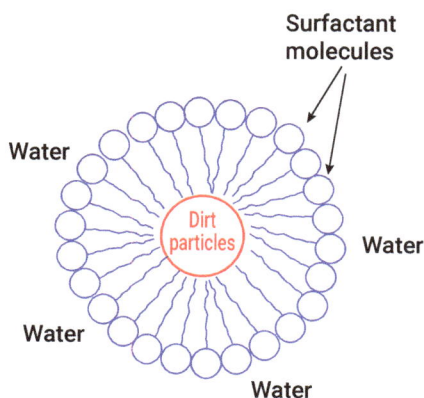

Figure IV-1-1. Solubilizing (dissolving) effect of surfactants: a contaminant particle coated with surfactant molecules in aqueous medium

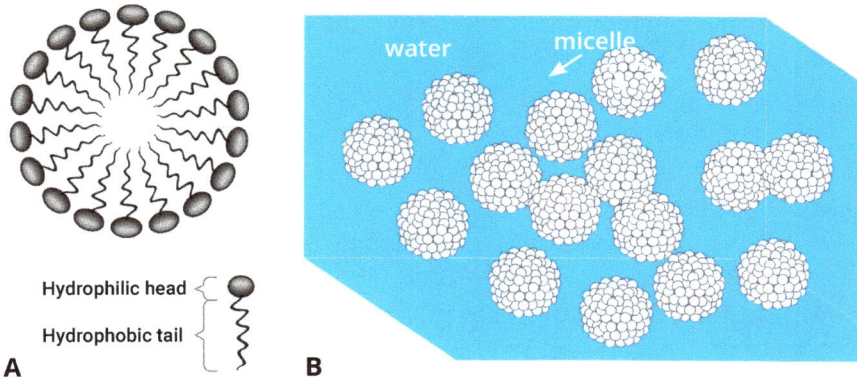

Figure IV-1-2. Micelle: A — structure; B — schematic of a micellar solution showing spherical micelles distributed in water (solvent) (Image by Wikipedia)

Micelle is an aggregate (or supramolecular assembly) of surfactant amphipathic lipid molecules dispersed in a liquid, forming a colloidal suspension (also known as associated colloidal system). A typical micelle in water forms an aggregate with the hydrophilic "head" regions in contact with surrounding solvent, sequestering the hydrophobic single-tail regions in the micelle centre. The micelle diameter ranges from 1 to 100 nm.

non-ionic surfactants). Cationic surfactants are the most dangerous for the skin, and are hardly ever used in modern skincare products.

In emulsions, surfactants are concentrated at the boundary of two immiscible phases — water and oil, forming a boundary monolayer which prevents droplet coalescence and phase separation. In solution, surfactants can form micelles (derived from Latin *mica* — particle, grain) (**Fig. IV-1-2**).

Anionic surfactants are characterized by good foaming and cleansing efficacy but can cause skin irritation and tightness. Therefore, to reduce the irritating potential of the finished product, they are combined with mild surfactants and/or conditioning agents. The mildest anionic surfactants are:

- Acyl phosphates (synthetic)
- Acyl sarcosinate (synthetic)
- Acyl taurates (synthetic)
- Isethionates
- Sulfoacetates

The following anionic surfactants should also be **avoided**:

- Alkyl sulfates
- Lauryl sulfates (sodium lauryl sulfate, ammonium lauryl sulfate, triethanolamine lauryl sulfate)
- Olefin sulfates
- Salts of fatty acids (soap)
- Alkyl aryl sulfonates (the most dangerous)

Amphoteric surfactants are milder than anionic surfactants, but their pH can vary considerably, due to which they are usually used as conditioning additives.

Non-ionic surfactants are the mildest surfactants that tend to suppress foaming. They are included in products aimed at children and those with severely damaged skin.

The most common mild surfactants (amphoteric and non-ionic) are:

- Alkylated amino acids
- Alkylamines
- Cocamidopropyl betaine
- Sodium lauroamphoacetate
- Sodium cocoamphopropionate
- Cocoaminopropionic acid
- Sodium lauraminopropionate
- Polyoxyethylated fatty alcohols
- Polyoxyethylated sorbitol esters
- Alkanolamides
- Poloxamer
- Alkyl glycosides

Surfactants vary widely in their irritant properties, which are mainly determined by their ability to bind to skin proteins and the depth of their penetration into the *stratum corneum*. Anionic (negatively charged) sulfate-based surfactants with short hydrophobic tails have the greatest irritant effect. These include sodium lauryl sulfate, a goldstandard irritant (as we have already mentioned, scientists usually use it in experiments to initiate skin irritation). However, the severity of the irritant effect of anionic and short-chain surfactants correlates with their concentration in the formulation and other ingredients, such as glycerol or betaines.

Since the irritant potential of a cleanser is determined by the surfactant composition, choosing these substances is particularly important when formulating a cleanser for sensitive skin with a weak or impaired barrier function. This is not an easy task, as most mild surfactants either do not form a good foam, do not give a sufficiently stable foam, or simply do not have the best cleansing power. One solution to this problem is to combine anionic sulfates (which can irritate the skin) with milder surfactants and betaines, thus lowering the concentration, and therefore the irritating potential, of the basic surfactants while still providing a good stable foam. An esterified version of anionic surfactants is also often used, which has a longer "tail" and is less damaging to the skin.

At the beginning of the 21st century, a group of particularly mild surfactants based on amino acids was launched in the cosmetics market. Along with good foaming properties, they do not damage the skin and are even moisturizing. Representatives of this category of surfactants are sodium cocoyl glutamate and sodium lauroyl oat amino acids.

The danger of surfactants for sensitive skin and/or skin with compromised barrier properties stems from their ability to penetrate the lipid barrier, embed themselves in it, and further disorder its structure. Therefore, traditional liquid or bar soap should be replaced by surfactant-free **micellar solutions** — suspensions of lipid micelles in water (see **Fig. IV-1-2**). When applied to the skin, the lipids embed themselves into the fatty plaques on the skin surface and crush them. Of course, the micellar solution will never exhibit the soap's effectiveness, which has a powerful cleansing action due to the presence of surfactants. Still, it is preferred for very sensitive skin, as its regular use does cleanse the skin, even if not as well as surfactants. That said, it is important to remember that **micellar solution must also be rinsed off like other cleansers**.

Low-viscosity emulsion, usually called **cosmetic milk**, is suitable for cleansing sensitive skin. It is worth bearing in mind that the milk also contains surfactants, as they are always present even in the most diluted emulsions. But if sensitive skin is quite heavily polluted, it is better to wipe it with milk and leave the micellar solution for cleansing not very polluted skin.

Finally, **syndets** are synthetic detergents with a pH of 5.6–6.5 and should be reserved for very dirty skin. Note: **regardless of the degree of contamination of the damaging skin, you cannot use traditional soap because it is alkaline!**

Today, new cleansers that also contain surfactants but are gentler to the skin are being developed by the cosmetic industry. Introducing such "gentle" surfactants makes it possible to bring the pH to the right range without harming the epidermal barrier.

Another factor to consider is how well the detergent rinses off the skin. Many problems are caused by substances that remain on the skin surface, which then slowly migrate into its deeper layers. If you have sensitive skin, you should only use products that can be easily removed by rinsing with water.

The irritating potential of a cleanser is modulated (up and down) by some other ingredients. Thus, the risk of irritation can be increased by fragrances and dyes and reduced by moisturizing agents (**Table IV-1-1**). A combination of several surfactants may make a product milder than an alternative based on a single surfactant. On the other hand, proteins, resins, and polymeric components may also reduce its irritant potential.

Table IV-1-1. Components of cosmetic preparations for skin cleansing

SUBSTANCE	FUNCTION	PRODUCTS
Water	• Dissolves and washes away dirt • Moisturizes and softens the skin • In the composition of the cosmetic product, it forms an aqueous phase in which the water-soluble substances present in the formulation are dissolved	Liquid soaps, gels, solutions, emulsions
Surfactants (anionic, amphoteric, non-ionic)	As a detergent: crush hydrophobic deposits on the skin surface, resulting in a suspension of microparticles in water that can be easily rinsed off	Natural and synthetic soaps
	As an emulsifier: stabilizes the emulsion, preventing its separation	Emulsions, scrubs
	As a foaming agent: when combined with water, forms a cleaning foam that emulsifies grease	Natural and synthetic soaps; foams and self-foaming emulsions

Continued on p. 83

SUBSTANCE	FUNCTION	PRODUCTS
Moisturizers (glycerin, polyquaternium-7, polyquaternium-10, chitosan)	Restore the water level in the *stratum corneum* and maintain its barrier properties	Emulsion-based products, oil-free water-based products, synthetic soaps
Skin conditioners (proteins, amphoteric surfactants)	Reduce the irritant potential	Liquid detergents, emulsions, scrubs
Viscosity regulators (polyols)	Adjust the viscosity of the finished product	Liquid detergents
Fillers (talc, kaolin, sodium silicate)	Prevent lumpy soap from soaking through	Bar soap
Preservatives	Prevent the microbial growth in the product and its biological decomposition	Emulsion-based, oil-free, water-based products
Fragrances	Mask the odor of other compounds and give the product its own pleasant aroma	All types of cosmetic products
Dyes	Color the product	All types of cosmetic products
Antibacterial agents	Inhibit the growth of microorganisms	Include products with claimed antibacterial properties: • for cleansing acne-prone skin (benzoyl peroxide) • for oily skin care (sulfur) • antibacterial soap (triclosan, triclocarban)
Exfoliating agents (hydroxy acids, abrasives)	Help soften and remove horny build-up. Designed for the care of skin with hyperkeratosis	• Glycolic and lactic acid in emulsion-based preparations, solutions (lotions) • Abrasives as a part of scrubs

1.3.2. Active additives

Moisturizers

Many modern cleansing formulations include substances that help to temporarily "lock" moisture on the skin surface, preventing its rapid evaporation (and hence the feeling of tightness), as well as bind to the *stratum corneum*, keeping it soft and flexible and preventing its cracking. Such additives are particularly important for industrial skin cleansers, as they significantly eliminate the discomfort caused by harsh surfactants and solvents. The same is true for baby wash and cleansing products, which are often applied onto damaged or irritated skin. These products have limited use in professional cosmetic treatments because they can leave a film on the skin, making it difficult for active ingredients to penetrate. However, they can reduce the risk of irritation in individuals with dry and sensitive skin.

The most common moisturizing ingredient in cleansing formulations is glycerin, while most frequently used moisturizing additives are mineral oil, amino acids, minerals, aloe gel, proteins, fatty alcohols (stearyl alcohol), propylene glycol, waxes, silicones (dimethicone), and natural oils.

Calming agents

Since many adverse post-washing reactions are caused by signaling molecules released from keratinocytes, skin immunocytes, or nerve endings, using plant extracts with bioactive substances that block inflammation can prevent or alleviate reactions such as itching, redness, and tingling. For this purpose, various additives are included in the formulation, which may include extracts of white willow, plantain, elderberry, algae, aloe, sea buckthorn, calendula, and other plants.

1.3.3. Peculiarities of using cleansers for sensitive skin

The cleanser should be applied with fingertips by gentle circular motions without rubbing or stretching the skin. It is also important to minimize the duration of contact between the cleanser and the skin. After soaping, the skin should be rinsed very thoroughly with warm water, as cold and hot water can provoke symptoms of sensitivity. If the skin reacts to water at any temperature, a cream-based cleanser should be removed with soft tissue. After washing, the skin should be blotted with a coarse-pile cotton towel or a paper towel. **Rubbing sensitive skin is not allowed!**

In cases of severe pollution, the soap solution should never be rubbed into the skin for a long time. It is better to soap the skin once more and then rinse it quickly.

Another thing to remember is that skin permeability increases after exposure to water, and the longer the exposure, the greater this change (a wet compress is the easiest way to increase skin penetration). If you apply creams and serums to such skin, more active substances will enter the deep layers, but will also facilitate the entry of auxiliary substances, which can be triggers of skin sensitivity. Therefore, it is generally better to wait until the skin is dry before applying care products.

1.3.4. Selection of cleanser

As mentioned previously, skin sensitivity can develop in people with low-sebum dry skin (more often) and with normal or increased sebum production. Therefore, the choice of a cleansing product should be made based on the sebum level. If the sebum production is excessive, a non-soap cleanser that does not contain fatty acid salts (no more than 10% of these substances are allowed) is recommended. If the skin produces an insufficient amount of sebum, products in the form of a light emulsion (cosmetic milk) with emollients are preferable. In all cases, without exception, the pH of the cleanser should be slightly acidic while remaining within the physiological pH range — i.e., it should be no higher than 5.5.

- **Normal skin or skin with a tendency towards dryness.** For skin with a normal or slightly reduced level of sebum, cosmetic milk specifically formulated for skin with a damaged barrier or a micellar solution can be used. However, while cosmetic milk can be removed with sponges, **micellar solutions must be rinsed off the skin**. Such soft cleansing base of emulsions, as a rule, can be enriched with soothing and calming extracts (e.g., calendula, rose, mallow) and softening components (e.g., apricot kernel oil, glycerin).

- **Dry skin.** Those with low-sebum skin should use mild soap-free cleansers based on micellar solutions or cosmetic milk free of traditional surfactants and alcohol, containing anti-inflammatory substances (plant extracts of chamomile, arnica, calendula, aloe, etc.). A creamy, low-foaming, and soap-free cleanser may be the optimal choice, as it not only cleanses but also moisturizes the skin.
- **Oily skin.** To cleanse the skin with excessive sebum, products with surfactants can be used. However, they should be non-aggressive (gels, foams) and should never be rubbed into the skin and left on the face for a long time. This is essential as, if contaminants are not completely removed with one application, it better to soap/rinse off several times. In addition, when scaling oily skin, products with salicylic acid can be used, but skin tolerance to these products should be evaluated individually.

1.4. Peeling the sensitive skin

People with sensitive skin are strongly discouraged from performing microdermabrasion and brushing, as well as from using loofahs, rough towels, scrubs, and other products that can damage the *stratum corneum*.

They should also refrain from acid and retinol peels, as acids can cause neurogenic inflammation, and retinol can lead to the thinning of the already thin *stratum corneum*, so the skin will react even more actively to the triggers.

However, mild exfoliation treatment is necessary as it stimulates epidermal renewal, including the renewal of damaged barrier structures.

Enzymatic peeling (exfoliation) is indicated for people with sensitive skin and pronounced irregularities of the *stratum corneum*. Enzymatic peels do not have a chemical irritating effect like products with AHA, and do not exhibit a mechanical irritating effect like scrubs. Moreover, enzymatic peels fit perfectly into the physiological skincare paradigm, mimicking the natural mechanisms of skin exfoliation.

Several proteolytic enzymes capable of breaking down proteins are found in the *stratum corneum*, but two serine proteases — chymotrypsin-like and trypsin-like — play the leading role in the exfoliation process. One of the reasons for slowing down the renewal of the *stratum corneum* is a decrease in the activity of proteolytic enzymes that destroy the corneodesmosomes. As a result, conglomerates consisting of horny masses, sebum, and impurities accumulate on the skin surface, which makes it dull and grayish in appearance.

Unlike AHA — which do not have any direct destructive potential, as they act indirectly by changing the pH gradient — the action of proteolytic enzymes is based on destruction. As they hydrolyze corneodesmosomal proteins, they can be denoted as keratolytic substances (substances denaturing proteins of the *stratum corneum*). Still, it should be noted that the action of enzymes is selective, as they exclusively destroy corneodesmosomes. This makes them fundamentally different from phenol, trichloracetic acid (TCA), and even salicylic acid, which non-selectively break intra- and intermolecular bonds of any proteins, causing their denaturation and destruction.

Enzymatic preparations are the only category of cosmetic products in which the presence of enzymes is at least biologically appropriate. Proteolytic enzymes "work" on the surface of the skin, whereby they loosen the adhesion of corneocytes by breaking the structural chemical bonds of corneodesmosomes, facilitating the exfoliation of horny scales. We emphasize that such cosmetic formulations were initially created to maintain enzymatic activity, not to "push" them deep into the skin.

The most common enzymatic peels include plant-based proteolytic enzymes such as papain, bromelain, and ficin. These enzymes belong to the cysteine proteases, having the amino acid cysteine in the active center. In addition, the papain and bromelain fractions have some lipolytic activity.

Papain is a hydrolytic enzyme found in all parts (except the roots) of the melon tree (*Carica papaya*), but the highest papain activity is found in the unripe green fruit. The papain content in papaya milky juice depends on the conditions in which the tree grew: the most favorable regions are those where humidity and solar activity are consistent throughout the year.

Bromelain is the common name for enzymes found in various plants of the *Bromeliaceae* family. It is a mixture of eight high-molecular-weight glycoproteins — cysteine proteases. Although bromelain from pineapple stems is the most extensively studied, some of these enzymes are present in leaves and fruits (green and ripe).

Modern preparations of enzymatic peels use **ficin** (obtained from the milky juice of fig tree *Ficuscarica*), **actinidain** (from kiwi), and **aleurain** (from barley), as well as proteases of mango, pumpkin, yam, and other plants.

Subtilisin (INCI: Subtilisin, Subtilopeptidase), a serine protease of microbial origin, is increasingly being incorporated into cosmetic formulations. It is produced by fermentation, akin to the process used in brewing. The U.S. Food and Drug Administration (FDA) has approved subtilisin as a safe enzyme suitable for human consumption. Because subtilisin is non-toxic, it is used in the production of cookies, candy, crackers, and laundry detergent. Subtilisin breaks more types of protein bonds than papain and is, therefore, more effective in breaking down protein deposits. A few years ago, Shiseido developed a polymerized subtilisin, which, according to the Shiseido researchers, is safer than the subtilisin monomer because it is less likely to penetrate the skin.

Different strains of *Bacillus subtilis* and some other microorganisms are used to produce subtilisin. The technologies of enzyme isolation, purification, and stabilization will also vary from one manufacturer to another (Karlsson C. et al., 2007). Therefore, the enzyme products obtained as the output do not share the same properties. Each manufacturer assigns a unique trade name to their product to distinguish it from its analogs. However, it is not yet a ready-to-use product, but rather a raw material, which is further included in the composition of finished cosmetic products. For example, an enzyme product called Travase® already available on the market is added to topical medications for clearing scabs from wounds (such preparations are used in burn therapy). Keratoline® is another subtilisin-based product adapted for use in cosmetics. It contains subtilisin dissolved in a liquid aqueous gel, while a small amount of glycerin and propylene glycol is added to stabilize the enzyme and facilitate its introduction into the cosmetic formulation.

Unlike other keratolytic peels (salicylic peel, Jessner peel), for which sebum deficiency is a contraindication, **the skin oiliness does not matter for enzymatic peels, which can thus be used at any level of sebum activity**.

Contraindications for enzymatic peels are atopic dermatitis and psoriasis. These pathologies are characterized by an increase in surface pH, which leads to a decrease in the activity of protease inhibitors in the *stratum corneum*. Accordingly, the activity of proteases increases, desquamation is intensified, and the *stratum corneum* becomes even thinner.

In addition, enzymes are proteins, and proteins are potential allergens. Given that immune dysfunction is involved in the pathogenesis of atopic dermatitis, the risks of an allergic reaction to a foreign protein are higher in those with sensitive skin than in healthy individuals.

In general, as with other cosmetic products, **people with sensitive skin are strongly advised to pre-test all products to determine individual reactions to them**.

When more aggressive peels are applied, the nature of the nervous reaction is such that the first response is usually the most intense. Then, habituation sets in, and the effect no longer elicits such a violent response. However, too strong or too frequent stimulation of free nerve endings can lead to hyperactivation of the sensory skin receptors, whereby response to weak stimulation generates disproportionately strong nerve impulses. The exposure that previously elicited only a sensory response then becomes the cause of neurogenic inflammation, and skin hypersensitivity occurs.

With repeated application of cosmetic products that irritate the C-fibers, two scenarios are possible. The first, favorable, involves desensitization (loss of sensitivity) of the nerve, whereby the level of reactivity decreases. For example, the skin becomes accustomed to the effects of acids if it is "accustomed" to gradually increasing the concentration, starting with a small "friendly" one.

Still, a less attractive course of events is also possible, where the nerve fiber response goes "off the scale." In this case, the nerve fiber releases signal molecules that affect immune cells and provoke inflammation. Then, instead of invisible skin irritation, which is felt only by the person complaining of itching, the real inflammation develops, accompanied by obvious external signs. As inflammation induces histamine release, itching is intensified, and edema develops due to increased vascular permeability. If the person starts to scratch the skin, this irritates the nerve endings and the itching increases.

It is worth noting here that, in many cases, the goal of a cosmetic procedure is to manage inflammation to stimulate skin remodeling. In this case, the depth and degree of traumatic effect are determined by the appearance and color of the skin. In invisible skin irritation, the patient begins to experience extreme discomfort long before the skincare practitioner notices any changes. With continued aggression and emergence of visible signs, inflammation can get out of control and, instead of positive changes, it may cause rashes, pigmentation, severe swelling, persistent irritation, etc.

It thus follows that any procedure on hypersensitive skin must avoid aggressive exposure because if a certain threshold of sensitivity is exceeded, the procedure can lead to uncontrolled inflammation.

At the same time, the potential for habituation, or desensitization, of the nerve fiber may allow a careful gradual action by which sensitivity can be reduced and the restoration of the skin barrier function can begin.

Chapter 2
Sensitive skin treatment

The next stage of sensitive skin therapy aims to influence different aspects of pathogenesis such as the skin barrier, sensory perception, and inflammation. In this context, qualitatively conducted diagnosis will help in the selection of the most optimal treatment options for a particular patient.

When diagnosing sensitive skin syndrome, it is important to acknowledge that it does not only affect the face. The skincare specialist must keep this in mind when recommending treatment: it is important that the client not only uses the right cream for the face, but also chooses appropriate products for hands, feet, hair, etc.

2.1. Restoring and maintaining the skin barrier

The skin barrier function is provided by many components listed in **Table IV-2-1**.

Table IV-2-1. Basic components of the epidermal barrier and their functions

COMPONENT	FUNCTION	LOCALIZATION
Corneocyte	Strength, stiffness, and impermeability of the *stratum corneum*	*Stratum corneum*
Corneodesmosomes	Ensuring the integrity of the *stratum corneum*	Between the corneocytes
Granular keratinocytes	Source of filaggrin and other NMF precursors, lipid barrier lipids, and *stratum corneum* enzymes	Boundary between granular and horny layers

Continued on p. 92

COMPONENT	FUNCTION	LOCALIZATION
Lipid barrier	Regulation of diffusion of substances through the *stratum corneum*, including water	Multilamellar lipid sheets between the corneocytes
Lamellar bodies (Odland bodies)	Source of lipid precursors that make up the lipid barrier	Boundary between granular and horny layers
Enzymes of the *stratum corneum*	Synthesis of extracellular lipids of the *stratum corneum*, desquamation of corneocytes	Inside the lamellar bodies, the *stratum corneum*
Natural moisturizing factor (NMF)	Water retention in the *stratum corneum*	Corneocytes, extracellular space of the *stratum corneum*
pH and Ca^{2+} gradient	Control of keratinization, secretion of lipid precursors of the lipid barrier, and enzyme activity within the *stratum corneum*	*Stratum corneum*
Hydrolipid mantle	Maintaining the microbiome, protection, providing a pH gradient trough the *stratum corneum*	Skin surface
Microbiome	Protection against pathogenic microorganisms, maintenance of skin barrier function, utilization of excretory products	Skin surface and appendages

With cosmetic products, we can influence the skin's metabolism and bring in substances from the outside that will strengthen the barrier, including the lipids.

Among skin surface lipids, two fractions that differ in the origin, composition, and properties are distinguished:

1. **Barrier lipids** are located in the *stratum corneum* between the corneocytes and form multilayer structure.
2. **Sebum lipids** are part of the hydrolipid acid mantle that covers the skin from the outside.

The barrier lipid composition of healthy skin is rather stable, and primarily consists of **ceramides (Cer), cholesterol (Chol), and free fatty acids (FFA)** in equimolar amounts (i.e., one molecule of cholesterol and free fatty acid per molecule of ceramides). The barrier lipids composition in wt% that corresponds to the equimolar ratio is shown in **Table IV-2-2**.

Table IV-2-2. Barrier lipids composition

LIPID SPECIES	wt%
Ceramides	40–50
Cholesterol	20–25
Cholesterol sulfate	5–10
Free fatty acids	15–20

The equimolar ratio of 1:1:1 is the most physiologic and provides good barrier function of the *stratum corneum*. However, this ratio will vary depending on the localization of the skin area and its thickness, as well as age, gender, race, health, and even climatic conditions (Yang L. et al., 1995).

Thus, to ensure the structural integrity of the *stratum corneum*, not only the qualitative composition but also the balanced ratio of its main components is important.

The lipid layers of the *stratum corneum* are positioned parallel to each other and are separated by a thin water layer through which water molecules move toward the surface: this process is called **transepidermal water loss (TEWL)**. When the structure of the lipid barrier is impaired, water movement is facilitated, and water begins to evaporate more intensively. The integrity of the lipid barrier ensures that water evaporation is controlled, that the hydration level of the *stratum corneum* is maintained at normal levels, and that foreign substances are prevented from entering the body.

Additional protection is provided by sebum consisting of refractory lipids: triglycerides (mainly), wax esters, squalene, and some free fatty acids, as shown in **Table IV-2-3**.

Table IV-2-3. Lipid composition of the hydrolipid mantle

LIPID SPECIES	wt, %
Triglycerides	42
Free fatty acids	15
Wax esters	25
Squalene	15
Cholesterol esters	2
Cholesterol	1
Vitamin E	<1
Carotenoids	<1

On the skin surface, sebum mixes with sweat and transepidermal water to form a **hydrolipidic mantle**. Covering the skin, it protects against pollution, softens the *stratum corneum*, reduces water loss, and controls microbiome. At the same time, oxygen and carbon dioxide pass through the hydrolipidic mantle quite freely. Sebum deficiency thus contributes to the development of dryness and increased skin irritability.

Since almost any type of sensitive skin involves impairment of the *stratum corneum* and water loss, when treating this condition, the aim is to restore the barrier structures and hydration of the *stratum corneum* (Snatchfold J., 2019).

2.1.1. Substances that restore the lipid barrier

These include essential fatty acids and physiological lipids in lamellar emulsions, liposomes, and nanocapsules. A physiologic combination comprising 1 (Cer — ceramide) / 1 (Chol — cholesterol) / 1 (FFA — free fatty acids) is considered optimal. For atopic dermatitis and some other skin diseases, the recommended formulation is 3 (Cer) / 1 (Chol) / 1 (FFA). In unbalanced diet and photodamage, the 1 (Cer) / 1 (Chol) / 3 (FFA) ratio is preferable. Skincare products with this lipid composition lead to the fastest recovery of barrier function, regardless of whether a concentrated or diluted lipid mixture is used.

Another option is to use natural oils as a lipid source, given that they do not contain any extraneous chemicals and are rich in phytosterols, vitamin E, and carotenoids referred to as biologically active substances.

However, they should still be used in moderation, given that the integrity of the lipid layers of the *stratum corneum* is maintained by the exact ratio of all lipid species (Cer / Chol / FFA). Plant oils are a mixture of triglycerides at their core. Although they can be enzymatically broken down into their constituent parts with the release of free fatty acids, they must first penetrate the lipid layers. If there is too much oil, it will dilute the lipid layers, temporarily disordering their structure. Usually, the structure of the *stratum corneum* is restored within a few days. However, too abundant and too frequent application of oils can lead to a permanent disruption of the skin's barrier function.

Avocado, rosehip, kukui nut, wheat germ, blackcurrant, evening primrose, and borage oils are the most physiologic in their chemical composition. The last three are especially valuable because, in addition to essential linoleic and linolenic acids, they contain γ-linolenic acid, a source of prostaglandin (PG) 1, which has a strong anti-inflammatory effect.

As natural oils are usually found in small amounts in cosmetic products, they do not affect the barrier structure as noticeably.

2.1.2. Homeostasis-stabilizing peptides

This group of peptides improves skin condition by activating its protective potential, affecting various skin structures from the *stratum corneum* barrier to the dermal matrix. Their well-known representative is the copper-containing peptide GHK-Cu (INCI: Prezatide Copper Acetate).

2.1.3. Pre- and probiotics

The current recommendation is to use cosmetics that are friendly to the skin microbiome. A healthy microbiome not only protects the skin from pathogens but also helps maintain skin barrier functions (Prescott S.L. et al., 2017). The following types of cosmetic ingredients are used for this purpose:

- **Probiotics** — active substances obtained from probiotic microorganisms that, when used in sufficient quantities, have a positive effect on human health.

- **Prebiotics** — substances (nutrition medium) needed for a healthy microbiome to function.
- **Synbiotics** — a combination of pre- and probiotics.

It is quite difficult to introduce **probiotics** into the composition of cosmetic products, as it is necessary to provide conditions for preserving their vitality while preventing the reproduction of "undesirable" microorganisms. One of the solutions to this challenge is the introduction of not whole bacteria but their fragments — lysates (fermented microorganisms), shells, enzymes, and DNA hydrolysates. These compounds interact with the receptors of skin cells, enhancing local immunity and producing anti-inflammatory factors. Some of them can be nutrients for other bacteria, i.e., prebiotics.

The use of **prebiotics** is also not without its challenges, as it has cost scientists a lot of effort to create a "nutrient base" that stimulates saprophytic bacteria but not pathogenic and opportunistic microflora. Typical prebiotics includes inulin, fructooligosaccharides, galactooligosaccharides, and lactulose. These have gradually been supplemented with xylooligosaccharides, long-chain β-glucans, and glucomannan.

Examples of **synbiotics** include these most frequently used combinations:
- Inulin + *Lactobacillus*
- Xylooligosaccharides + *Lactobacillus*, *Streptococcus*, and *Bifidobacterium*
- Lactosucrose + *Lactobacillus* and *Bifidobacterium*

The effectiveness of pre- and probiotics in treating skin pathologies has been extensively studied and the obtained results are impressive. For example, research findings show that topical application of cream with *Lactobacillus plantarum* on acne-prone skin helps to reduce the number of inflammatory papules and pustules and erythema. *Vitreoscilla filiformis* lysate application reduces inflammation and significantly improves atopic and seborrheic skin conditions compared to placebo (Muizzuddin N. et al., 2012, Mottin V.H.M., Suyenaga E.S., 2018).

A cream with *Bifidobacterium longum* extract was shown by Guéniche A. et al. (2010) to lower the reactivity of sensitive skin in clinical trials. Since *B. longum* lysate has been shown to inhibit capsaicin-triggered CGRP release and improve barrier function, these authors hypothesized that the reduction in skin sensitivity was due to a combination of suppressed neuronal reactivity and decreased neuronal availability to stimuli through barrier strengthening.

There are also reports that glucooligosaccharides can be successfully used to control *Staphylococcus aureus* in atopic skin (Blanchet-Réthoré S. et al., 2017). Moreover, various formulations with β-glucans have been shown to improve wound healing and reduce skin dryness and itching in bacterial infections (Kiousi D.E. et al., 2019).

An important aspect of the action of topical probiotics is their ability to maintain surface pH within the normal range. The same is true for **acidotherapy** remedies, as applying acidified products to the skin can significantly improve its barrier function.

2.1.4. Special diet

It is important to ensure the body gets enough fats to build a strong protective barrier, as well as micronutrients and antioxidants. Special nutritional supplements (nutraceuticals) containing omega-3/6 poly-unsaturated fatty acids, carotenoids, vitamins C, E, and D, and plant antioxidants belonging to the group of polyphenols can help to balance the diet.

2.2. Skin moisturizing

2.2.1. Occlusion and artificial hydrolipid mantle

The occlusive and sebum-like ingredients create an artificial semi-permeable film that will prevent water evaporation from the skin and increase the hydration of the *stratum corneum*. The sebum acts as a natural occlusive film, as oxygen and carbon dioxide pass freely through it, and water evaporation is inhibited due to glycerin it contains and by the smoothing of horny scales. Glycerin holds water molecules by electrostatic forces. It also has a mild "enveloping" effect that reduces the sensitivity of nerve endings. As a result, some cosmetic ingredients mimic sebum in order to slow down water evaporation, including:

- Mineral oil, vaseline, liquid paraffin, ceresin: hydrocarbons, petroleum products
- Liquid silicones (silicone oils): hydrophobic high-molecular-weight organosilicon compounds
- Lanolin: an animal wax obtained from the purification of wool wax
- Animal fats: goose fat, whale (spermaceti) fat, pork fat, badger fat
- Squalene and its derivate squalane: a natural component of human sebum obtained from shark liver and some plants
- Vegetable oils: mostly solid oils, such as shea butter (karite oil)
- Natural waxes and their esters: beeswax, vegetable waxes (pine wax, cane wax, etc.)

2.2.2. Water saturation of the *stratum corneum* from within

To increase the water-holding potential of the *stratum corneum*, hygroscopic substances that attract and hold water molecules due to the presence of charged groups are used.

These substances are divided into two groups according to their molecular weight:
1) high-molecular-weight compounds
2) low-molecular-weight compounds

High-molecular-weight molecules (> 3000 Da) cannot penetrate through the *stratum corneum* and remain on its surface, forming a kind of "wet compress" on the skin. They include:

- Natural polysaccharides: hyaluronic acid, chondroitin sulfate, pectins, etc.
- Proteins of animal and plant origin and their hydrolyzates: collagen, elastin, keratin, chitosan
- Polynucleic acids (DNA) and their hydrolysates

This group also includes propylene glycols, but their use is not recommended for hypersensitive skin (Aravijskaya E.R., 2008).

Deep moisturizing of the skin is provided by the NMF — a complex of low-molecular-weight hygroscopic substances normally found within the *stratum corneum*. Thus, NMF components contained in cosmetic products are beneficial for dry and dehydrated skin. Hygroscopic moisturizers include the following substances commonly found in topical products:

- Urea (however, it has irritant potential)
- Amino acids
- Lactic acid and sodium lactate
- Sodium pyroglutamate
- Glycerin
- Sorbitol trioleate
- Glyceret-26
- Methylglucet-2
- Sorbic acid

Unlike high-molecular-weight compounds that remain on the skin surface, NMF components pass into the *stratum corneum* and increase its water-holding potential from within (thus achieving so-called "deep moisturizing"). The moisturization that is felt in this way is usually not as pronounced and does not come on as quickly as the "wet compress" effect, but it lasts longer and is less dependent on the air humidity.

2.3. Decreasing excitability of the skin receptors

Not many agents that can affect TRP channels are known. However, developments in this field are underway. The following agents that can bind to TRPV receptors and reduce their sensitivity to triggers are presently used:

- Defensol Soft (INCI: *Albatrellus Ovinus* Extract)
- Skinasensyl (INCI: Acetyl Tatrapeptide-15)
- Rhamnosoft HP 1.5 P (INCI: Biosaccharide Gum-2)
- Trans-4-tert-butylcyclohexanol (INCI: 4-tert-Butylcyclohexyl Alkohol)
- Delisens (INCI: Acetyl Hexapeptide-46)

The activity of some of these compounds is very high. For example, just two molecules of grifolin, one of the active components of northern truffle, provide a complete blockade of one TRPV1 receptor. Moreover, it has been shown that the extract reduces sensitivity to all TRPV1 triggers — heat, capsaicin, and others (Hettwer S. et al., 2017).

In any skin sensitivity, a normalizing effect on the psycho-emotional sphere is highly beneficial and can be achieved by the following practices:

- **Use of cosmetic products with a pleasant texture and cold creams that soothe the skin.** It is better to replace "heavy" creams containing petrolatum, paraffin, and mineral oil with "lighter" silicone-based creams.
- **Relaxing massage** with a soothing gentle action on the skin receptors. Even for the routine application of cosmetic products, it is recommended to use a massage that will address specific acupuncture points.
- **Relaxation practices** such as yoga, breathing exercises, meditation, and autotraining.
- **Physical activity.** During exercise, there is a release of endorphins, "happy hormones" with anti-inflammatory activity.
- **Psychological assistance** ranging from counseling by appropriate specialists to creating a relaxing atmosphere in the treatment room and beauty salon. For this purpose, various techniques can be used to affect the different sense receptors, including olfactory (aromatherapy, but it is necessary to avoid sharp smells and contact of components with the skin), auditory (music therapy), and visual (color therapy).
- **Physical therapy,** e.g., aerotherapy, halotherapy, cryosauna, etc.

2.4. Anti-inflammatory measures

Another important goal of sensitive skin therapy is the inhibition of inflammation (including neurogenic inflammation). The following substances can help to achieve this aim:

- **Plant extracts with soothing and anti-inflammatory effects**: centella, chamomile, white willow, raspberry, aloe juice, plantain, etc.

- **Immunomodulatory peptides** to normalize the immune status of the skin. These include Rigin tetrapeptide (INCI: Palmytoyl Tetrapeptide-3), which restores cytokine balance, reduces inflammation and improves skin condition.
- **Neurotransmitter peptides** affect the cutaneous nerve endings, reducing skin sensitivity to environmental factors. They are modified enkephalins or stimulate enkephalin release in the body. These so-called "feel-good peptides" include Calmosensine (INCI: N-Acetyl-Tyrosyl-Arginyl-Hexadecyl Ester) and Leuphasyl (INCI: Water (and) Glycerin (and) Pentapeptide-18 (and) Caprylyl Glycol).
- **Thermal water** with minerals and trace elements with anti-inflammatory properties.
- **Physiotherapeutic treatments**, such as bubble baths, galvanization, and low-level laser (light) therapy (LLLT). The LLLT effect was confirmed in a study conducted by Korean scientists, whereby 630-nm laser energy was used to treat sensitive skin in 30 patients with ≥ 40 Misery scale scores. The twice-weekly sessions performed for eight weeks reduced the symptom severity by 60% in 93% of the participants (Sonbol H. et al., 2020).

The use of antioxidants is also recommended for individuals with sensitive skin because all inflammatory processes are accompanied in one way or another by a release of reactive oxygen species. Their generation is also triggered by UV light and air pollutants.

Popular antioxidants include:
- Vitamin C
- Vitamin E
- β-Carotene
- α-Lipoic acid (thioctic acid)
- Coenzyme Q_{10} (ubiquinone)
- *Maritime pine* bark extract
- Green tea extract
- Acai berry extract
- *Polypodium leucotomos* fern extract
- *Centella asiatica* extract
- Boswellia extract
- Resveratrol

- Tranexamic acid
- Lactobionic acid

Many of these compounds have not only antioxidant but also anti-inflammatory and soothing effects.

2.5. Peculiarities of care for atopic sensitive skin

As previously mentioned, surface lipids are an essential part of the epidermal barrier, and are divided into two fractions:
1) **sebum lipids** on the skin surface
2) **extracellular lipids** between the horny scales

The sources, composition, and functions of these two lipid fractions differ, but their joint contribution to the maintenance of the protective function of the *stratum corneum* is exclusive. If, for any reason, there is a lipid imbalance, it immediately reduces its barrier potential, as confirmed in patients with atopic dermatitis.

Defective DNA loci responsible for the maturation of the *stratum corneum* in atopic dermatitis have already been identified, and the specific molecular mechanisms in which the malfunctions occur have been elucidated. As shown in **Tables IV-2-4** and **IV-2-5**, genetically determined changes affect both lipid fractions, explaining why the skin of atopic patients is always dry and low in sebum and why its protective properties are reduced.

The renowned dermatologist Peter Elias, a student of Albert Kligman and one of the founders of corneotherapy, suggested correcting lipid imbalances by applying special topical preparations that specifically restore and maintain the barrier function of the skin (Elias P.M., 2010). "Ordinary" emollients and moisturizers which differ in their mechanism of action and should be selected according to skin conditions are unsuitable for this purpose. According to Elias P.M. (2018), a skincare product (or several products) for an atopic patient (with a confirmed diagnosis) should simultaneously "work" on the following three fronts:

Table IV-2-4. Sebum composition alteration in atopic skin

LIPID SPECIES	HEALTHY SKIN $\mu g/cm^2$	ATOPIC SKIN $\mu g/cm^2$	CHANGES
Squalene	12.8 ± 0.6	10.8 ± 1.1*	↓
Cholesterol	1.2 ± 0.2	2.4 ± 0.4*	↑
Cholesterol esters	1.3 ± 0.2	2.4 ± 0.6*	↑
Wax esters	25.6 ± 3.2	21.7 ± 1.8*	↓
Triglycerides	36.1 ± 8.4	32.6 ± 10.6	downward trend
Free fatty acids	21.6 ± 8.8	28.8 ± 11.4	upward trend
Diglycerides	1.4 ± 0.2	1.3 ± 0.2	no changes
TOTAL	**195.4 ± 20.6**	**172.6 ± 17.4**	↓

* Statistically significant compared to healthy skin, $p < 0.05$.

Table IV-2-5. The *stratum corneum* alterations in in atopic skin

INTERCELLULAR LIPID STRUCTURES	CORNEO-DESMOSONES	HORNY SCALES
Alterations in the activity of enzymes responsible for lipid structures assembly result in changes in lipid composition: • ↓ Ceramides • ↓ Sphingosine • ↓ Free fatty acids • ↓ Cholesterol • ↓ Cholesterol sulfate	Increased activity of proteolytic enzymes destroying corneodesmosomes	Mutations in genes that inhibit the maturation of filaggrin and loricrin result in: • Corneocytes shape changes • ↓ NMF (sodium pyro-glutamate, urocanic acid, free amino acids)
↑ TEWL	Severe exfoliation	↓ Hydration

1) like sebum, serve as a surface emollient and create an additional protective coating
2) correct the imbalance of extracellular lipids to restore and maintain the barrier function
3) moisturize the skin (especially in severe xerosis), providing a "wet compress" effect

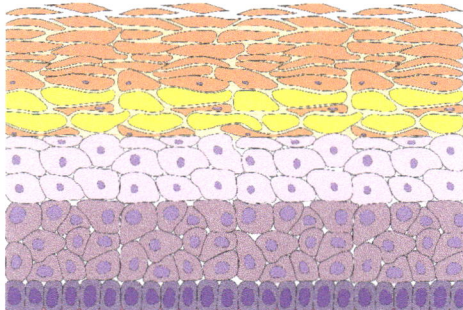

3. Imitation of sebum: ointments
Vaseline, high-molecular-weight silicone oils, refractory fats, squalene

2. Wet compress (for pronounced dryness, if necessary)
Lamellar emulsions, glycerin, hygroscopic polymers (PEG, hyaluronic acid, etc.)

1. Restoration of the intercellular lipid barrier
Ceramides, unsaturated fatty acids, cholesterol

pH 5.0–5.5

Therapy aim:
prolong the remission by strengthening the barrier structures

Figure IV-2-1. Lipid replacement topical therapy (numbers indicate the order of application)

Fig. IV-2-1 shows a scheme of application of cosmetic products with different mechanisms of action to replenish lipids and water in the *stratum corneum* of atopic skin.

Special ingredients will ensure that these tasks are carried out effectively. We want to draw special attention to the fact that these ingredients are not drugs with restrictions on their use. They are all used in cosmetic products in one way or another (considered as substances that form the product's base, not as active agents) and do not have undesirable side-effects like steroids. Still, to provide the necessary triple effect, it is important to choose the right combination as well as correct proportions of these ingredients within the formulation.

Another important point is to ensure that the pH of the preparation is about 5.5 (atopic people tend to be somewhat alkaline, so it is important to keep the redox balance on the skin surface within the normal range).

According to this strategy, Dr. Elias developed EpiCeram® Skin Barrier Emulsion, approved in 2006 by the FDA for patients with atopic dermatitis. The following components are responsible for accomplishing the three main tasks:

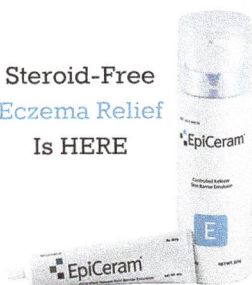

Steroid-Free
Eczema Relief
Is HERE

Imitation of sebum — squalene, dimethicone, candelilla wax, capric acid, glyceryl stearate, petroleum jelly, palmitic acid

Correction of the composition of extracellular lipids — cholesterol, conjugated linoleic acid, ceramides

"Wet compress" — cornstarch, glycerin, PEG-100 stearate, xanthan gum, water

Once EpiCeram® entered the market, it became the prototype for a new generation of preparations that restore and strengthen the barrier properties of the skin in atopic dermatitis. Subsequent cosmetic formulations are based on the framework formulation proposed by Dr. Elias, although they differ in the sebum-like vegetable oils with high density (such as shea butter), waxes, or silicone oils). The preparations include substances that reduce inflammation and itching (nicotinamide). Finally, great attention is paid to the base. After all, aesthetics — pleasant texture, lack of stickiness and greasy shine, etc. — is an essential aspect of all cosmetic products. In terms of these properties, silicone oils are superior to organic oils; in addition, silicones are biologically inert and resistant to oxidation and photodegradation, which makes them an excellent base for cosmetics. Another option is to use lamellar emulsions, which are prepared without traditional surfactants and are much gentler on the skin.

In pharmacies, you can now find cosmetic lines designed for comprehensive care of skin with impaired barrier function, from hygienic cleansing to restoration and protection. Pharmaceutical companies are also actively exploring this field and, along with medicines, are investing into the production of special cosmetics designed to help patients relieve unpleasant sensations (e.g., itching, skin tightness) during the manifestation of the disease and to prolong remission.

It is very important for atopic patients to treat their skin carefully and not provoke its damage, given that the weakened skin barrier is a peculiarity with which they must learn to live, and the "right" cosmetic products can significantly help them to do so.

Part V

Age-related changes in skin sensitivity

Chapter 1
Epidermal function

As we age, the skin changes not only in appearance but also in functionality. Many people who had no special problems with the skin begin to complain about its increased irritability in older age, including inadequate reaction to cold and hot temperatures, rashes after washing, unpleasant subjective sensations (feeling of tightness, itching), and so on. Those who have experienced dermatologic problems (atopic dermatitis, seborrheic dermatitis, infectious lesions, etc.) may notice their exacerbation.

Behind the external and functional alterations, there are changes in the structure of skin tissues. However, the problem of high sensitivity is primarily related to changes at the epidermis level because this is where the main defense mechanisms of the skin are localized.

Fig. V-1-1 summarizes all the major epidermal changes observed with aging (Wang Z. et al., 2020) described in detail in the sections that follow.

1.1. Barrier function alterations

The barrier function of the *stratum corneum* is assessed by measuring TEWL, which increases dramatically when the barrier is compromised.

In intact skin, mean normal TEWL values vary depending on gender, part of the body, and skin pigmentation. Although the correlation between TEWL and age is insufficiently explored, available data show that average TEWL values on some body parts in older people may be lower than in younger individuals (Boireau-Adamezyk E. et al., 2014), indicating the more reliable barrier in older skin. However, there is

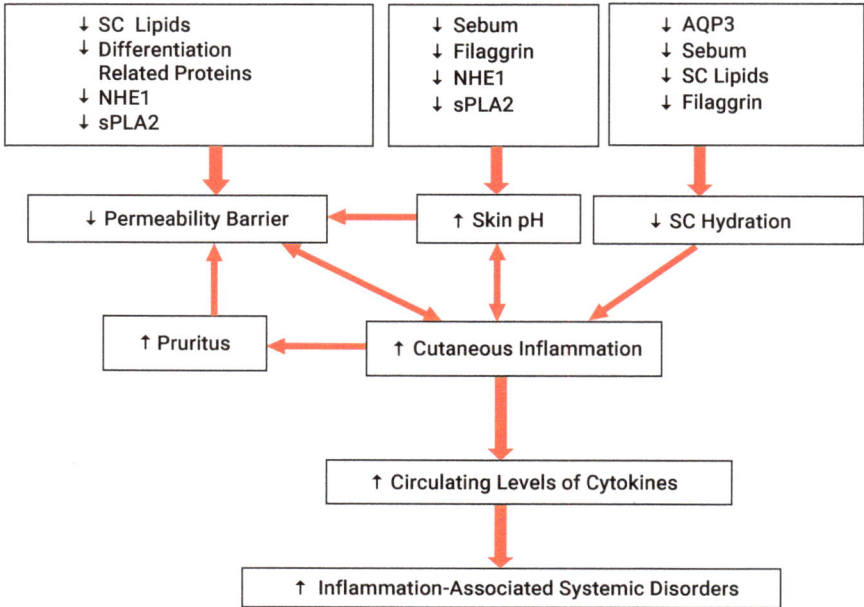

Figure V-1-1. Aging associated changes in epidermal function and their clinical significance (adapted from Wang Z. et al., 2020)

an age-related increase in TEWL in the décolletage area, suggesting the opposite. On the neck, forearms, and hands, young and older women have comparable TEWL levels (Luebberding S. et al., 2013a). TEWL is also higher on average in older women than in older men (Luebberding S. et al., 2013b).

Despite the scattered results, one thing is clear: the TEWL levels in healthy, intact skin of people of different ages, although slightly different, are not so critical to speak about the pathological disturbance of the barrier function during aging. However, there is still an age-related problem: after damage to the *stratum corneum*, the restoration of barrier function in elderly people is much slower than in younger individuals due to the biochemical and structural changes in the epidermis that occur with age.

Recall that the skin permeability barrier is localized in the *stratum corneum*. It consists of keratin-filled corneocytes surrounded by a cornified envelope made of proteins and alternating lipid and water layers between the corneocytes regulating the diffusion of low-molecular-weight substances through the *stratum corneum*. The functioning of the barrier is largely determined by the quantity and quality of protein and lipid substances formed during the maturation of keratinocytes and their final transformation into corneocytes.

1.1.1. Epidermal growth factor

In the epidermis of aging skin, the level of epidermal growth factor decreases along with a decline in the basal keratinocyte division rate. At the same time, the number of keratinocyte apoptoses increases. All these processes lead to the thinning of both living layers of the epidermis and the *stratum corneum* (Gilhar A. et al., 2004; Kinn P.M. et al., 2015).

1.1.2. Calcium ion concentration gradient

With age, there is a change in the Ca^{2+} gradient in the epidermis, another important factor controlling the division and maturation of keratinocytes and the formation of the *stratum corneum*. Thus, in the basal and spiny layers of the epidermis of elderly people, Ca^{2+} concentration is higher, which inhibits keratinocyte proliferation (Denda M. et al., 2003; Micallef L. at al., 2009).

In contrast, in the granular layer, Ca^{2+} levels fall, and this impairs the maturation of *stratum corneum* proteins (filaggrin, loricrin, etc.) (Takahashi M., Tezuka T., 2004; Rinnerthaler M. et al., 2013), which can lead to the formation of defective corneocytes and alterations in the permeability barrier (Scharschmidt T.C. et al., 2009).

1.1.3. Extracellular lipid sheets of the *stratum corneum* (lipid barrier)

Extracellular lipid layers also exhibit age-related changes. The formation of lipid barrier requires cholesterol, free fatty acids, and ceramides in approximately equal molar ratios (Man M.Q. et al., 1996). These lipids are synthesized by keratinocytes, and deficiency in any of them can lead to defects in barrier structures (Feingold K.R., Elias P.M.,

2014). Studies have shown that the "old" *stratum corneum* has >30% lower total lipid content compared to the "young" *stratum corneum* (Ghadially R. et al., 1995), which is associated with a decrease in the synthetic activity of keratinocytes both in the intact and injured skin. Thus, applying a mixture of barrier lipids can improve barrier function in the elderly, which confirms the presence of age-related barrier dysfunction (Zettersten E.M. et al., 1997).

1.1.4. pH gradient across the *stratum corneum*

One of the stages of lipid barrier formation is the enzymatic transformation of lipid precursors into barrier lipids. This transformation is already carried out outside keratinocytes in the extracellular spaces of the *stratum corneum* (Man M.Q. et al., 1995). Besides enzymes responsible for the lipid barrier, there are enzymes in the *stratum corneum* that ensure the timely desquamation of horny scales by breaking down corneodesmosomes (proteolytic enzymes). All these enzymes, like any other enzymes, are very sensitive to the pH level. There is a pH gradient in the *stratum corneum*, from an acidic value of about 5.5 (the hydrolipid mantle on the skin surface) to a slightly alkaline value of about 7.2 (at the border with the granular layer). Thus, different layers of the *stratum corneum* will have distinct pH levels, controlling the enzyme activity at a certain depth (**Fig. V-1-2**).

With age, surface pH tends to increase (Choi E.H. et al., 2007; Man M.Q. et al., 2009; Schreml S. et al., 2012), which changes the pH gradient across the *stratum corneum*, and this affects enzyme activity. Specifically, proteolytic enzymes in the middle and on the top of the *stratum corneum* are activated at higher pH, which accelerates exfoliation. In contrast, enzymes responsible for the lipid barrier are depressed at higher pH, resulting in an altered lipid barrier. All these processes combine to weaken the permeability barrier of the *stratum corneum* (**Fig. V-1-3** and **V-1-4**).

Application of preparations with neutral pH delays barrier repair; in contrast, acidification of the *stratum corneum* accelerates barrier repair in both young and aging skin (Hachem J.P., 2003; Choi E.H. et al., 2007; Hachem J.P. et al., 2010).

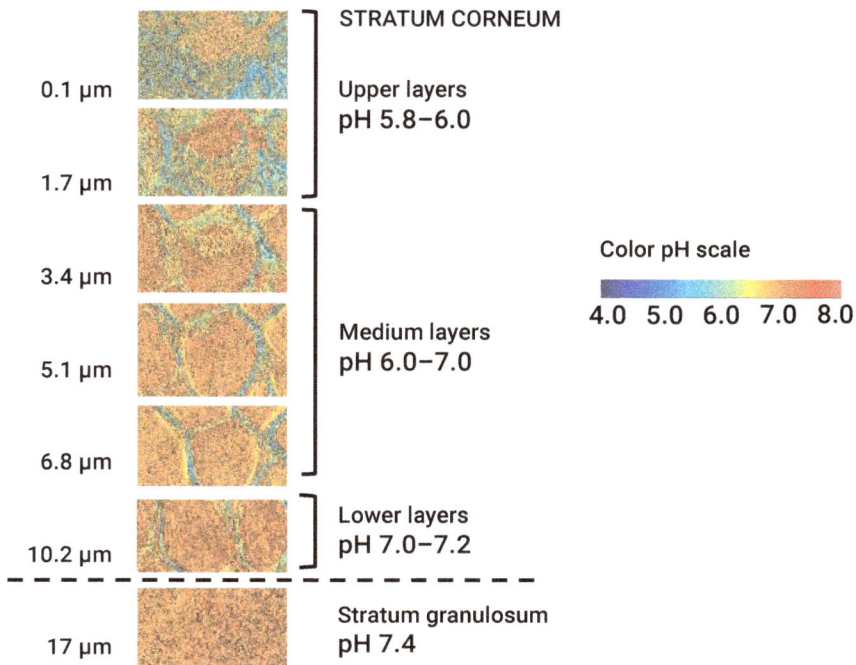

STRATUM CORNEUM

0.1 µm

Upper layers
pH 5.8–6.0

1.7 µm

3.4 µm

5.1 µm

Medium layers
pH 6.0–7.0

6.8 µm

Color pH scale

4.0   5.0   6.0   7.0   8.0

10.2 µm

Lower layers
pH 7.0–7.2

17 µm

Stratum granulosum
pH 7.4

Figure V-1-2. pH gradient across the *stratum corneum*: assessment by two-photon spectroscopy (adapted from Hanson K.M. et al., 2002)

Special molecules, so-called fluorescent probes, are applied to the skin. They penetrate the *stratum corneum* and, upon further irradiation with light of a certain wavelength, become excited and release excess energy in photons. This secondary emission is called fluorescence and can be recorded. To determine the pH of the *stratum corneum*, a probe was chosen that can emit in both acidic and alkaline environments, but this emission will be at different wavelengths. In the resulting image, the luminescence in an acidic environment is indicated in blue and in a neutral-alkaline environment in orange. The obtained color images can be used to calculate the average pH at different depths of the *stratum corneum* based on the ratio of blue to orange areas.

The closer to the surface, the bluer the color. The calculated average pH in the upper layers of the *stratum corneum* is slightly higher than in the hydrolipid mantle but is still acidic — less than 7.0. In the middle of the *stratum corneum*, the pH approaches neutral values, and it becomes progressively more alkaline at further depths.

Color distribution in the *stratum corneum* is uneven, as indicated by clearly demarcated blue (acidic) and orange (neutral) areas. The *stratum corneum* consists of dense, almost water-free horny scales, within which the pH is neutral. Free water in the *stratum corneum* is in the extracellular space, and this, too, as clearly shown here, will be acidified.

That is, even in the lowest layers of the *stratum corneum* we still see areas with acidic pH, although there are fewer of them. But under the *stratum corneum*, water is found both in the cells and in the extracellular space. As the pH here is slightly alkaline, we do not see individual cells but a uniform orange coloring.

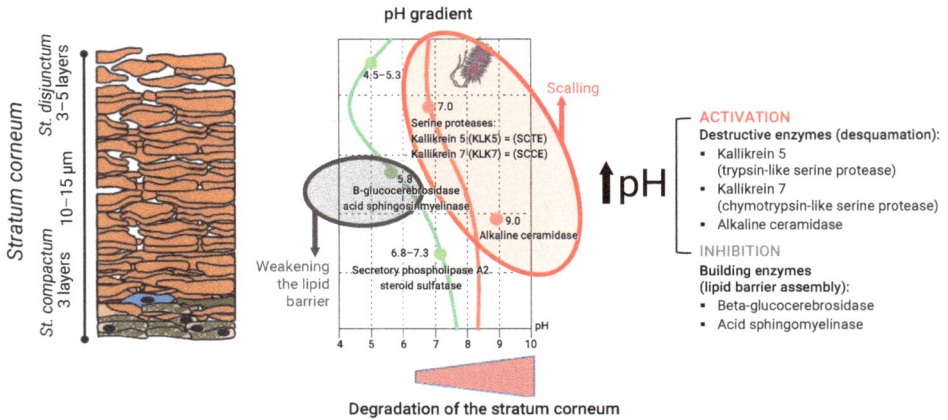

Figure V-1-3. An increase in surface pH modulates the pH gradient across the *stratum corneum* and results in enzymatic activity alterations

As the pH value increases, enzymes responsible for lipid barrier assembly are inhibited, leading to the formation of desordered lipid layers and the weakening of the permeability barrier. Conversely, proteolytic enzymes that degrade corneodesmosomes are activated, resulting in increased desquamation and visible scaling.

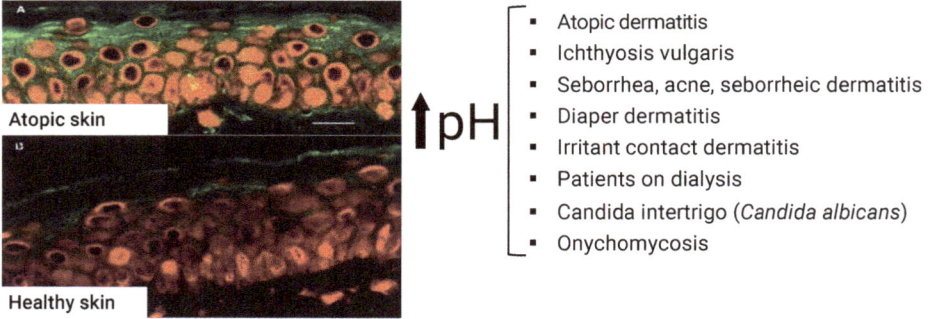

- Atopic dermatitis
- Ichthyosis vulgaris
- Seborrhea, acne, seborrheic dermatitis
- Diaper dermatitis
- Irritant contact dermatitis
- Patients on dialysis
- Candida intertrigo (*Candida albicans*)
- Onychomycosis

Increased serine protease activity in atopic dermatitis (top) compared to normal (bottom) skin. Orange fluorescence correlates to serine protease activity. Contributed by Dr. Peter Elias (unpublishd data) (Ali S.M., Yosipovich G., 2013)

Figure V-1-4. Skin pathologies associated with elevated surface pH

1.1.5. Glucocorticoids and cortisol

Biological aging is accompanied by increased glucocorticoid and cortisol levels in the skin (Yiallouris A. et al., 2019). Studies have shown that systemic or topical application of glucocorticoids inhibits keratinocyte proliferation and weakens the barrier (Kao J.S. et al., 2003). In the skin, cortisone is converted to its active form, cortisol, by 11β-hydroxysteroid dehydrogenase 1 (Tomlinson J.W. et al., 2004). In aging skin, the activity of this enzyme increases (Tiganescu A. et al., 2011), and this negatively affects the epidermis' ability to repair and form a barrier (Choe S.J. et al., 2018). Inhibition of 11β-hydroxysteroid dehydrogenase 1 not only corrects glucocorticoid-induced epidermal functional impairment but also promotes the restoration of barrier structure (Tiganescu A. et al., 2013; Tiganescu A. et al., 2018).

1.1.6. Other factors

Other factors associated with skin aging may contribute to alterations in epidermal function. For example, compared to the young epidermis, IL-1 receptor antagonist levels in the aging epidermis decline by >60%, and IL-1α type 1 receptor deficiency delays barrier repair (Ye J. et al., 2002). In contrast, increased expression and administration of IL-1α strengthen the barrier in both aging and fetal skin (Barland C.O. et al., 2004; Jiang Y.J. et al., 2009).

Aging also leads to a **decrease in the hyaluronic acid** levels. Studies have shown that topical application of hyaluronic acid stimulates keratinocyte differentiation and lipid production, which increases the epidermal permeability barrier function in both young and aging skin (Bourguignon L.Y. et al., 2006; Bourguignon L.Y. et al., 2013).

Finally, **decreased expression of epidermal aquaporin-3** — a protein that forms water channels in the keratinocyte membrane and is responsible for extracellular water balance — is observed with age (Li J. et al., 2010; Ikarashi N. et al., 2017). Silencing the gene encoding aquaporin-3 delays permeability barrier repair (Hara M. et al., 2002). In contrast, enhancing aquaporin-3 expression improves barrier function (Schrader A. et al., 2012).

1.2. Decreasing hydration of the *stratum corneum*

In most individuals, the hydration level of the *stratum corneum* begins to decrease in the fifth decade of life. This phenomenon can be explained by a deficiency of substances in its water-regulating and water-retaining structures.

First, the total amount of barrier lipids (Ghadially R. et al., 1995; Rogers J. et al., 1996), including ceramides (Imokawa G. et al., 1991), decreases in the *stratum corneum* of aging skin. Their deficiency can be compensated by oral or topical application of ceramides, which leads to increased hydration of the *stratum corneum* (Huang H.C., Chang T.M., 2008; Bizot V. et al., 2017).

Second, levels of filaggrin (Takahashi M. et al., 2004) and its metabolites — including *trans*-urocanic and pyroglutamic acids, which are part of the natural moisturizing factor (NMF) — are reduced. Application of these substances, as well as other components of NMF, such as free amino acids, lactic acid, and urea, helps to increase hydration.

Third, the production of sebum, in general, and glycerol, in particular, is lower in aging skin than in young skin (Choi E.H. et al., 2005; Man M.Q. et al., 2009). Sebum, together with sweat, forms a hydrolipid mantle that regulates water evaporation from the skin. If the mantle is disturbed, evaporation increases. Thus, in low-sebum skin, there is a decrease in the hydration of the *stratum corneum*, and the application of preparations that mimic the hydrolipid mantle helps to restore it.

Finally, the level of aquaporin-3 decreases in the aging epidermis (Li J. et al., 2010; Schrader A. et al., 2012). This impairs the movement of water in the living layers of the epidermis and promotes the development of congestion, due to which the division and maturation of keratinocytes are inhibited. Aquaporin channels can be activated in the presence of a small amount of glycerol (a few percent) in the environment (Dumas M. et al., 2007); high concentrations of glycerol (over 10%), on the contrary, inhibit their work.

1.3. Increasing the pH of the skin surface

The pH value of the human skin surface tends to be higher in the first two weeks of life, decreasing to an average of 5.5 by weeks 5–6 (Fluhr J.W. et al., 2012). After the age of 55, skin surface pH tends to increase, and in people over 70, this increase becomes significant. Normal human skin surface pH values depend on gender and body part (Zlotogorski A., 1987).

The age-related increase in skin surface pH is due to several factors. One of them is a decrease in sebum production and, consequently, in the total amount of triglycerides, from which free fatty acids are released, acidifying the hydrolipid mantle and the surface of the *stratum corneum* (Yamamoto A. et al., 1987). In its lower layers, the *stratum corneum* is acidified by the release of free fatty acids from cell membrane phospholipids under the action of secretory phospholipase 2 (sPLA2) (Fluhr J.W. et al., 2001), the expression of which decreases markedly with age.

Another mechanism regulating the pH gradient in the *stratum corneum* involves the Na^+/H^+ exchanger-1 (NHE1): when NHE1 is deficient, skin surface pH increases (Behne M.J. et al., 2002). In aging skin, NHE1 expression is significantly lower than in young skin, which may contribute to an increase in surface pH.

Finally, aging skin shows low filaggrin expression levels, which can be cleaved to *trans*-urocanic acid via the filaggrin–histidine–urocanic acid pathway (Vávrová K. et al., 2014). Urocanic acid acidifies the *stratum corneum* (Krien P.M., Kermici M., 2000).

Chapter 2
Clinical implications of age-related changes in the epidermis

2.1. The impact of hypohydration of the *stratum corneum*

Reduced *stratum corneum* hydration is involved in the pathogenesis of senile xerosis and pruritus (Valdes-Rodriguez R. et al., 2015). In patients with such diagnoses, inflammatory infiltration, mast cell density, degranulation, and histamine levels in the dermal layer increase (Ashida Y., Denda M., 2003). Itching provokes scratching, resulting in damage to the *stratum corneum*, which, in turn, leads to a further increase in inflammation.

Because permeability barrier homeostasis in aging skin is disrupted, it cannot be rapidly normalized, leading to a persistent increase in skin inflammation and exacerbation of pre-existing inflammatory conditions such as atopic dermatitis and eczema. Continued worsening of skin inflammation may eventually lead to systemic inflammation and related diseases (Hu L. et al., 2017; Ye L. et al., 2019).

In addition, night itching can cause insomnia, contributing to the exacerbation of pathologies such as cardiovascular disease and Parkinson's disease (Bollu P.C., Sahota P., 2017).

2.2. The role of barrier function failure

The regeneration of *stratum corneum* barrier structures is slower in aging skin, although its barrier function in the absence of damage is comparable to that observed in young individuals. Various pathogens enter the skin through damage in the barrier, provoking an inflammatory response and itching (Lin T.K. et al., 2013), which can serve as a trigger for the exacerbation of atopic dermatitis (Tanei R., Hasegawa Y., 2016) or development of contact dermatitis (Prakash A.V., Davis M.D., 2010). Persistent cutaneous inflammation can trigger systemic inflammation, whereas defects in the permeability barrier promote bacterial colonization (Wanke I. et al., 2013; Jinnestål C.L. et al., 2014).

2.3. The role of pH changes

Increasing the skin surface pH alters the pH gradient across the *stratum corneum*, affecting the function of *stratum corneum* enzymes and the spatial configuration of protein and lipid species of the lipid barrier.

First, changes in extracellular lipid layers occur due to the disruption of enzymes responsible for lipid barrier formation (β-glucocerebrosidase, acid sphingomyelinase, secretory phospholipase A2). Accordingly, the permeability barrier of the *stratum corneum* is broken.

Second, the antimicrobial properties of the skin are altered (Korting H.C. et al., 1990) as acidic pH inhibits the activity of *Staphylococcus aureus* and fungi (Rippke F. et al., 2018). In individuals with increased pH, these and other pathogens begin to grow and can trigger the development of skin infections. Indeed, the incidence of skin infections increases with advancing age.

Third, the activity of proteolytic enzymes of the *stratum corneum*, responsible for exfoliation of the corneocytes, increases. As neutral and alkaline pH values are optimal for them, acidic pH restrains their activity at the necessary level (Jang H. et al., 2016). When pH rises, proteases cleave corneodesmosomes more actively, which leads to visible scaling and inflammation.

Chapter 3
Anti-ageing skincare and nutraceutical products for sensitive skin

Use of special topical and nutraceutical products can slow down the development of age-related epidermal dysfunction and correct existing disorders.

3.1. Acidification of the *stratum corneum* (acidotherapy)

Acidifying the *stratum corneum* may strengthen the barrier and improve its recovery from injury, as confirmed in several studies. For example, the application of lactobionic acid normalizes the homeostasis of the barrier and the structure of corneodesmosomes (Hachem J.P. et al., 2010). Kilic A. et al. (2019) also demonstrated that topical application of an emollient with pH 4.0 for 29 days in elderly people gives similar results, as their *stratum corneum* showed a marked increase in hydration, improved organization of lipid layers, and overall increased resistance to potential irritants such as sodium lauryl sulfate. The emollient at pH 4.0 has also been shown to accelerate barrier recovery from acute injury and to significantly improve *stratum corneum* integrity after 28-day treatment in elderly people compared to the emollient at pH 5.8 (Lee H.J. et al., 2017).

3.2. Topical application of barrier lipids

Applying a lipid mixture containing the three main lipids of the *stratum corneum* — Cer, Chol, and FFA — contributes to restoring the lipid barrier of aging skin (Denda M. et al., 1993). Moreover, topical application of an emollient containing barrier lipids not only strengthens barrier function, improves *stratum corneum* hydration, and normalizes surface pH, but also reduces levels of circulating pro-inflammatory cytokines in aging skin (Ye L. et al., 2019). There is an explanation for this phenomenon.

First, lipids penetrate the *stratum corneum* and reach granular keratinocytes. Keratinocytes capture and accumulate them in lamellar granules with special enzymes (Man M.Q. et al., 1993; Man M.Q. et al., 1995). Subsequently, the contents of lamellar granules spill out into the extracellular space, where the assembly of lipid layers begins under the control of enzymes.

Second, fatty acids included in topical lipid composition can activate peroxisome-proliferator-activated receptors (PPAR) of keratinocytes, thus stimulating synthesis of epidermal lipids and transformation of keratinocytes into corneocytes. As a result, the barrier is strengthened, and inflammatory processes are attenuated (Man M.Q. et al., 2006).

3.3. Other substances of natural origin

Epidermal function in the elderly can also be improved by some other substances in topical preparations but also those taken orally.

For example, food supplementation with vitamin C, linoleic acid, wheat oil extract, and borage oil reduces clinical signs of senile xerosis and strengthens the barrier function (Cosgrove M.C. et al., 2007; Guillou S. et al., 2011; Boisnic S. et al., 2019). Positive effects on epidermal function have also been shown in estrogen replacement therapy (Thornton M.J., 2013; Chen Y. et al., 2017).

Still, cosmetic products are the main care tool for aging skin issues, as they contain barrier lipids, antioxidants, and NMF substances as active agents. Lipids can be included into natural oils, especially blackcurrant, borage, evening primrose, coconut, and soybean oils (Vaughn A.R. et al., 2018). Extant research on the potential application of enzymes involved in forming lipid layers further shows that applying bacterial sphingomyelinase from *Streptococcus thermophiles* increases the hydration of the *stratum corneum* and its ceramide content in elderly people (Di Marzio L. et al., 2008).

When choosing cosmetic products, not only the active ingredients but also the substances in the base should be considered. For example, petroleum jelly and glycerin are useful for strengthening the barrier in elderly people. Vaseline mimics sebum — it adheres to the skin surface and restrains water evaporation (occlusive effect). Glycerin is a low-molecular-weight hygroscopic substance that penetrates the *stratum corneum* and works similarly to NMF substances, i.e., it binds water inside the s*tratum corneum*. In low concentrations, these substances have a beneficial effect on hydration and reduce skin reactivity. However, in high concentrations, negative effects can be observed. For example, too strong occlusion in the case of large amounts of petroleum jelly will lead to hyperhydration of the *stratum corneum*, making it less resistant to microbial invasion and more prone to infection. Glycerin, if taken in large quantities (more than 10%) and applied to the damaged barrier, will penetrate beneath the *stratum corneum* and may block the aquaporin channels of keratinocytes. Thus, these substances should not be considered inert and the importance of their concentration should be kept in mind when formulating skin-treatment products (Czarnowicki T. et al., 2016; Páyer E. et al., 2018).

In aging skin, multiple changes in epidermal function occur, which may contribute to the development of cutaneous and somatic pathologies. Therefore, improvement of epidermal function can be an effective method of prevention and treatment of these diseases.

Unfortunately, a significant proportion of topical products on the market claimed as "emollients" are not suitable for sensitive aging skin because they were not formulated with age-related structural and biochemical changes in mind (Huang Y.S. et al., 2011; Kwa M. et al., 2017; Huang L.N. et al., 2018). Such preparations often contain oils enriched with eicosanedioic acid, stearic acid, ceteareth 20, PEG-40 castor oil, and PEG-100 stearate, all of which, while softening the skin, can cause inflammation and/or disrupt the epidermal barrier.

In addition, acidification is indicated for aging skin, i.e., it benefits more from products with pH 4.0–5.0, not the "classic" 5.5 (sometimes you can find products with pH close to the neutral values, i.e., about 7.0, and their developers emphasize this as a virtue, although it is contrary to scientifically proven facts).

Such emollients, especially in the long term, may impair the epidermal functions, leading to the development and exacerbation of diseases associated with its dysfunction. Therefore, when choosing emollients, not only the product's composition but also its pH should be considered.

Part VI

Psychology:
skin hypersensitivity
as a manifestation of
a sensitized personality

In the skincare practice, some clients complain about their skin condition and adverse reaction to cosmetic products, but there are no objective cutaneous symptoms of skin hypersensitivity. Such people are quite emotional and convincing in their statements about the skin problems they experience. In most cases, the specialist gives recommendations, which do not always lead to the desired result, and may sometimes even provoke subjective symptom deterioration. Therefore, the client is rightfully dissatisfied. Is this the whim of a "fastidious client" or the cry for help of a "suffering patient"? In the latter case, what is the reason for the suffering? How can this person be helped? This is the topic of the current chapter.

From the point of view of medical psychology, the absence of objective symptoms with a variety of subjective manifestations testifies to the functional nature of the disorder. It suggests that the causes of this condition lie primarily in the psychic sphere of the patient's personality.

1.1. Relationship between a patient's mental state and skin condition

To begin, we need to recognize that a patient seeking help from a skincare specialist is a personality consisting of psyche and soma. This classification is confirmed by the holistic approach to studying personality, according to which "personality can only be understood as a holistic entity" (Hjell L., Ziegler D., 2009).

In addition, there is a close relationship between the patient's mental state and the state of his or her body, in particular, the skin

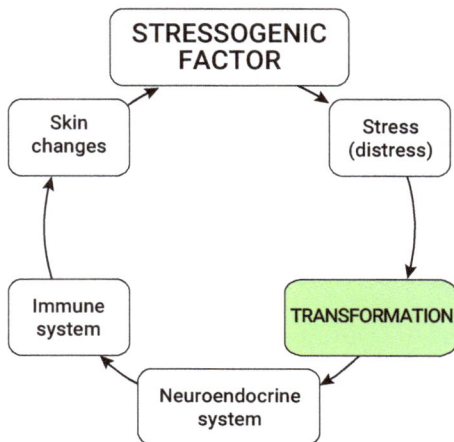

Figure VI-1-1. Interrelation of mental and somatic (in particular, skin) components of personality in a stressful situation: emotional tension is transformed into somatic symptoms

condition (**Fig. VI-1-1**) (Novitskaya N.N., 2015). This relationship becomes particularly pronounced in situations that are stressful for the individual (Nikolaeva N.N., 2017).

First, emotional stress is accompanied by the sympathoadrenal system activation which involves all organs and systems (including the skin). Under the influence of adrenaline, microcirculation is disturbed (narrowing of arterioles is observed), which leads to a violation of metabolic processes inside and outside the skin cells. Under the influence of cortisol, the barrier function of the skin is impaired, dryness appears, and the metabolic activity of fibroblasts is suppressed so that the production of hyaluronic acid, collagen, and other components of the dermal matrix is reduced. These processes create conditions conducive to infection and inflammation (Novitskaya N.N., 2009).

Second, emotional impact stimulates the release of histamine, proteases, and other biologically active substances in the skin, which leads to the formation and intensification of inflammatory reactions (Reilly D.M. et al., 2000). In addition, the skin perception function is violated by the increase in the receptor sensitivity to neurotransmitters (substance P) and the expression of nerve growth factor (NGF) (Baumann L., 2012; Kail-Goryachkina M.V., Belousova T.A., 2016).

Third, the skin plays an important role in psycho-neuroimmune interactions: it not only contains receptors for almost all neurotransmitters and hormones of the hypothalamic-pituitary-adrenocortical system but also produces them (Szepietowski J., Reich A., 2004). Besides, the skin participates in immune protection: nowadays, the skin is considered a lymphoepithelial organ providing lymphocytes with the optimal environment and conditions for immune response. All this allows us to conclude that the skin is an organ directly involved in the organism's reaction to stress.

The skin also performs several psychological functions:

- It is an integral part of the "I"-concept formation as the basis of personality.
- It plays an important role in creating an overall impression of a person (attractiveness).
- It participates in sensory cognition (skin is a huge receptor field through which information from the outside world arrives in the CNS, and sensations are formed).
- It performs a communicative function in the form of tactile interaction, which is especially important in childhood.
- It participates in the expression of emotions by changing color ("erythema of bashfulness," "turned white with fear," etc.).

All the above points to the fact that changes in the mental sphere of the personality will entail changes in the skin, and skin disorders will affect the mental state of the personality.

The skincare specialist thus needs to understand that a personality characteristic such as sensitivity pertains to the person, not just the skin.

1.2. The concept of sensitivity at the skin level and the personality level

As a part of their meta-analysis based on data obtained in 26 studies, Chen W. et al. (2020) established 71% global prevalence of "self-reported" sensitive skin syndrome in the adult population.

If we consider sensitivity as a skin condition, we can say that sensitive skin is one in which low tolerance to aggressive external influences due to the deterioration of protective and barrier mechanisms is combined with increased reactivity.

It should be noted that the concept of "sensitivity" exists not only in medicine but also in psychology. It is a characterological feature

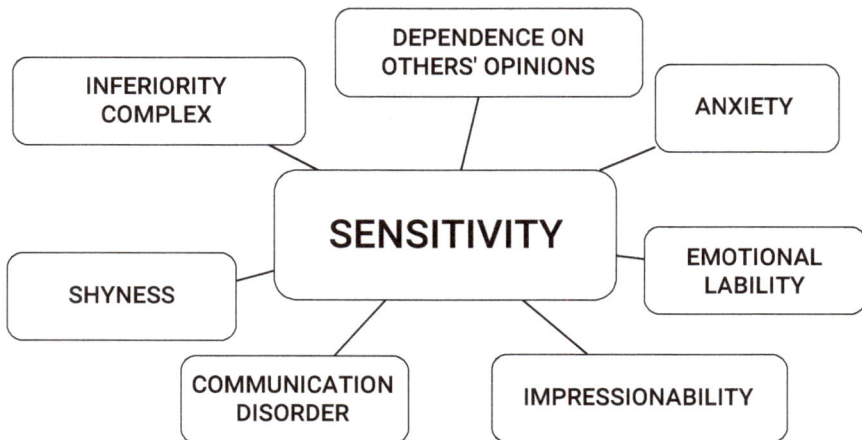

Figure VI-1-2. Psychological manifestations of personality sensitivity

of a person, manifested in increased sensitivity to events that occur to him/her usually accompanied by increased anxiety, fear of new situations, people, all kinds of tests, etc. (Petrovsky A.V., 1990). Sensitivity at the psychological level is manifested by heightened impressionability, anxiety, emotional lability, resentfulness, inferiority complex, low self-esteem, tendency toward exaggeration, communicative incompetence, etc. (**Fig. VI-1-2**). In this regard, the findings related to the psychology of patients with sensitive skin are of interest, as they indicate that skin hypersensitivity is correlated with somatic and phobic anxiety, hostility, and sensitivity in interpersonal relationships (Baumann L., 2012).

At the level of personality, sensitization is a set of psychosomatic symptoms based on low tolerance and increased reactivity to factors within the external and internal environment.

Sensitivity on a psychological level can be related to:

- Distress
- Accentuation (i.e., the reinforcement of character traits)
- Psychopaths
- Neurosis
- Mental illnesses (schizophrenia, etc.)
- Pre-morbid conditions

That is, sensitive skin can be seen as one of the manifestations of a sensitized personality at the biological level.

Many authors distinguish four levels in the personality structure:

1. Biological (the organism itself, including the skin)
2. Psychological (emotions, thinking, memory, character, etc.)
3. Social (roles in society, communication, etc.)
4. Spiritual (values, worldview)

Hence, at the biological level, personality sensitivity is manifested in the form of sensitive skin syndrome; at the psychological level, it is revealed in character traits (impressionable, anxious, with an inferiority complex, etc.). At the social level of the personality, the first place is occupied by a disturbance in communication (such people often yield to others to the detriment of their interests, are resentful, etc.), which, in turn, causes prolonged emotional tension that triggers somatic reactions (see **Fig. VI-1-1**). On the spiritual level, such people are often characterized by high morality, as well as the ability to be compassionate and empathetic.

In his book *Saying Yes to Life: a Psychologist in a Concentration Camp*, the famous Austrian psychotherapist, psychologist, and philosopher Viktor Frankl emphasizes that, paradoxically, sensitive individuals proved to be more resistant to abuse in the concentration camps. He attributed this phenomenon to the fact that such personalities, due to their subtle perception of the world, are capable of finding a unique meaning of life in a particular situation, which sustains them during hardships (Frankl W., 2019).

To understand how this is realized in practice, let us consider a clinical case.

1.3. How a skincare practitioner can become a psychologist

A patient came to the clinic complaining about her unsatisfactory skin condition (**Fig. VI-1-3**). She noted unpredictable skin reactions to various cosmetic products, discomfort, and skin tightness. "I am already afraid to put anything on my skin and can't go without cream," the patient specified during the first consultation.

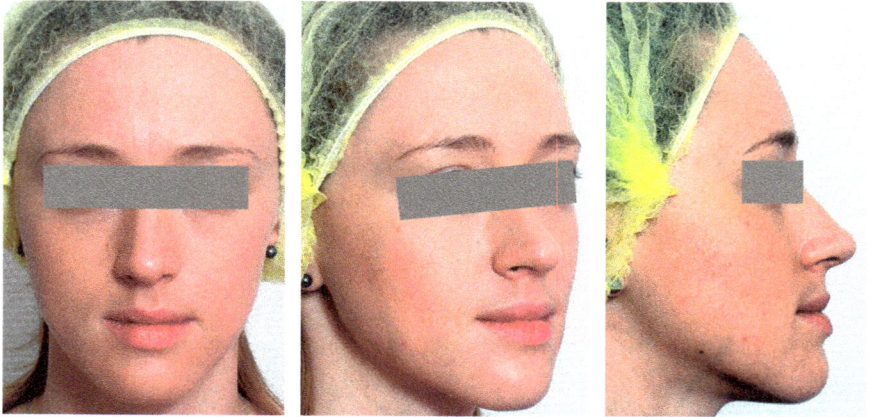

Figure VI-1-3. Patient A., 29-year-old woman with sensitive skin syndrome (Photo: Nikolaeva N.N.)

Yet, during objective examination, no visible changes in the skin were found. Dermatoscopy showed weakly expressed mucoid desquamation classified as type S3 "Burning and searing" according to Baumann's classification of sensitive skin types.

The patient was also tense, fearing for the skin condition, and fidgety.

With the patient's consent, the clinician administered the test for determining the type of personality accentuation (TTPA), which yielded the diagram shown in **Fig. VI-1-4** (note that, in the absence of abnormalities, the scales should be within the red lines).

TTPA conclusion

Individuals of this type are characterized by excessive reactivity and instability (lability) of emotional state, whereby even insignificant events cause mood downswings and upswings easily. Such people have low self-esteem, are anxious, pessimistic, restless, passive, timid, and shy, lack self-confidence, are impressionable, sensitive, resentful, reticent in social contacts, suspicious of everything new, and resistant to change. Getting stuck on negative experiences, they can be intemperate, irritable, irascible, and prone to verbal aggression (quarrels, insults, threats). Their aggressive, angry reactions are easy to arise, impulsive, and poorly controlled.

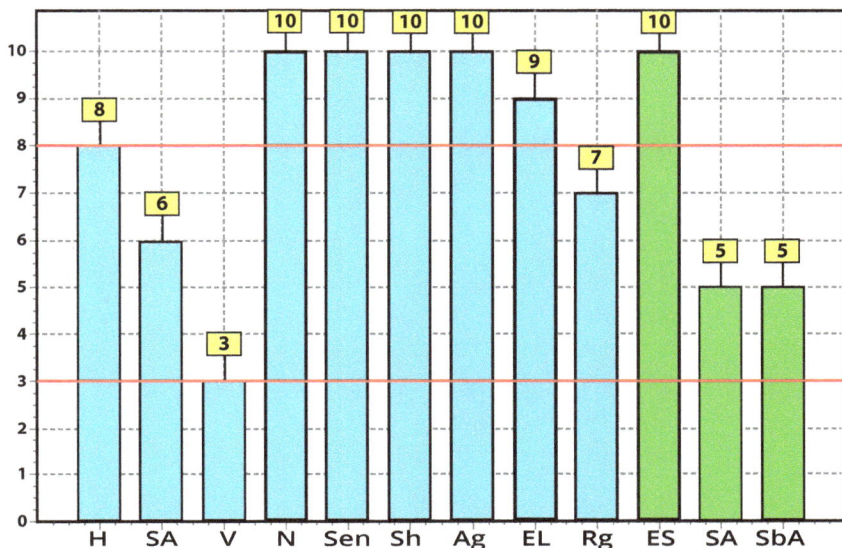

Figure VI-1-4. Patient A., TTPA results

Abbreviations: H — hyperthymia; SA — social activity; V — vigor; N — neuroticism; Sen — sensitivity; Sh — shyness; Ag — aggressiveness; EL — emotional lability; Rg — rigidity; ES — emotional stability; SbA — subject activity.

The test results were discussed with the patient and she agreed to a comprehensive therapy, including psychological correction and cosmetic procedures.

In this patient, we see signs of sensitivity both at the biological level (sensitive skin) and at the psychological level (based on the conversation and test results). Considering the peculiarities of her personality, we can assume difficulties in communication with other people (social level of personality).

Of course, help for such patients should be comprehensive, addressing all levels of personality. It is this personal approach to solving the problems of patients with sensitive skin that can provide the desired results and improve their quality of life.

Psychological correction should be aimed at relieving emotional tension, increasing psychological stability, changing the attitude towards oneself, and developing communication skills. Relaxation techniques, methods of rational psychotherapy, etc., are effective in this situation.

When providing skin therapy, in this case, it is better to perform care procedures using cosmetic products for sensitive skin and avoid aesthetic invasive methods that are damaging the skin barrier.

1.4. Complex treatment

Skin therapy for Patient A. included procedures using cosmetics for sensitive skin at intervals of 3–4 days. At the same time, the skincare therapist applied relaxation techniques.

During this procedure, the patient lies down on the couch so that she is comfortable while maximizing relaxation.

Cosmetic treatment is performed with successive application of cosmetic products, including a soothing mask.

Relaxation. The patient closes her eyes, regulates breathing with emphasis on exhalation (relaxation breathing), and mentally repeats phrases spoken by the skincare specialist (e.g., "I feel the muscles of the face, neck, etc. relaxing").

The treatment is completed by removing the soothing mask and applying a cream for sensitive skin.

In addition, the patient was interviewed using rational psychotherapy methods to break down her misconceptions about her condition through explanations and logical persuasion (e.g., to correct the patient's fears about her skin condition and possible reactions to applying cosmetics).

The intensive course lasted for two months, and upon its completion, the patient was given recommendations regarding home skincare regimen, including relaxation at least three times a day (the patient was previously trained in relaxation techniques). The patient visited the cosmetologist approximately once every 1.5–2 months. During these appointments, she underwent supportive cosmetic procedures using cosmetics for sensitive skin, as well as psychological correction.

A second intensive course of 8-week duration was conducted six months after the first. The patient has been under observation for about a year. She notes improved condition, as she is calmer and more self-confident, and has made new friends. The patient stopped giving excessive importance to her skin condition, and noted the absence of discomfort, calmly using the prescribed cosmetic products (**overly attentive attitude to the skin condition has decreased**). Objective examination confirmed absence of pathological changes in her skin; at dermatoscopy, there was no mucoid desquamation. But the most important thing is the patient's assessment of the treatment results: "I have no skin problems now."

As this example shows, sensitive skin is like the tip of an iceberg, the basis of which is a sensitized personality. Accordingly, therapy offered to patients with sensitive skin should combine psychological correction and cosmetic treatment.

Recommendations for a skincare specialist when working with a sensitive personality

- Timely diagnosis of sensitive personality (need to consult a psychologist, or psychiatrist)
- Combining psychological correction with cosmetic procedures
- In communication with such patients, criticism, value judgments, and displays of superiority should be avoided

Part VII

Sensitive scalp: diagnosis and treatment strategy

This book concludes with a separate discussion of the condition associated with scalp hypersensitivity. This problem can bother those with other manifestations of sensitive skin syndrome or can emerge as a separate complaint. In such cases, the help of a trichologist is not necessary, as a consultation with a qualified skincare specialist can significantly alleviate the client's condition.

Sensitive (reactive, hyperreactive) skin is a term widely used by clinicians, cosmetic manufacturers, and consumers. The condition is defined as subjective skin symptoms such as burning, burning, tingling, soreness, or itching provoked by exposure to various factors (Misery L. et al., 2008). According to the International Classification of Diseases 10 (ICD-10), sensitive skin syndrome can be coded as "Other and unspecified skin changes" (R23.8).

As the pathology of this condition is poorly understood, the term "sensitive skin" is frequently used in the context of intolerance of facial skin to cosmetics. Still, these unpleasant subjective symptoms may also be present on other body parts, especially hands, head, neck, torso, back, and genitals (in descending order of frequency of reports). Sensitive scalp syndrome appears to be part of the general sensitive skin syndrome, but the hyperreactivity may be limited to a single site. Hypo-diagnosis of the condition is typical. Subjective symptoms are difficult to assess objectively and may be transient, subtle, and external clinical manifestations may be variable or absent. As a result, the problem is underestimated by doctors as well as patients.

Skin hypersensitivity is rarely the main reason to consult a trichologist. Still, it is often a concomitant condition that complicates the treatment process (the selection of topical therapeutic agents in particular) and requires immediate attention. Although, at first glance, the pathology seems insignificant, specialists should attempt to identify it, as it is the cause of constant internal discomfort and irritable behavior of the patient.

A progressive course with the formation of intolerance to cosmetic products characterizes sensitive skin syndrome. To describe the condition of scalp hyperreactivity with loss of sensitivity to any external stimuli, including standard therapeutic measures, a new concept — **scalp burnout** —has been proposed. This name is analogous to the concept of emotional burnout, which is characterized by mental exhaustion and limited potential for recovery in later stages of development. Scalp burnout syndrome is not included in the ICD-10 nor is it a specific skin disease, but rather a common and difficult-to-diagnose and treat clinical condition.

Patients with scalp hypersensitivity often report concomitant hair loss (Misery L. et al., 2008). We hypothesize that trichodynia may be an aspect of the sensitive scalp syndrome. This condition (considered poly-etiologic) is defined as sensations of discomfort, soreness, and paresthesias on the scalp in patients with hair loss complaints. According to the available research findings, perifollicular inflammation, secretion of neurotransmitters (substance P), and concomitant psychiatric disorders may contribute to its formation (Willimann B., Trüeb R.M., 2002).

The problem of sensitive skin is widespread, given that 38.4–52% of the participants in large epidemiologic studies conducted in the UK, France, and the U.S. reported symptoms of facial skin hypersensitivity (Willis C.M. et al., 2001; Misery L. et al., 2009, 2011). Comparable figures were obtained in another large study about scalp hypersensitivity conducted in France. Based on 1,011 observations, the authors reported that it affected 47.4% of women and 40.8% of men (Misery L. et al., 2008).

1.1. Etiology and pathogenesis of sensitive scalp syndrome

Increased environmental and psycho-emotional load on modern people, as well as changes in lifestyle (primarily in megacities), contribute to the growing incidence of sensitive skin condition. Various internal and external factors can provoke this condition. Pathogenetically, the sensitive skin syndrome is caused by a decrease in skin tolerance to external influences combined with hyperreactivity, due to which it cannot normally perform its functions. In studies of biophysical parameters of sensitive skin, impaired skin barrier function was associated with increased TEWL and skin pH value (Seidenari S. et al., 1998). Compared to healthy skin, sensitive skin is more likely to have decreased elasticity, hydration, and external manifestations in erythema and telangiectasias (Seidenari S. et al., 1998).

The condition of skin hyperresponsiveness with the presence of multiple telangiectasias, which occurs against the background of topical application of glucocorticosteroids or antiseborrheic agents and is exacerbated by UV radiation, is described as a separate syndrome — **red scalp** (Trüeb R.M., 2014). Internal predisposing factors that impair skin tolerance may include (Misery L. et al., 2008):

- Physiologic age-related skin changes, especially senile asteatosis (from Greek, *a* — negative particle, *stear* — fat)
- Dermatologic diseases that lead to increased dryness and impaired desquamation (atopic dermatitis, ichthyosis, psoriasis)
- Hormonal disorders
- Psycho-emotional stress
- Systemic drugs (isotretinoin)

The irritant potential of the components of external products intended for regular scalp care (shampoos, conditioners, scrubs, and peels), products used in hairdressing procedures (coloring, permanent straightening, and perming), medications for the treatment of hair and scalp (e.g., alcohol-containing growth stimulators) should thus be considered. Disruption of the barrier function of the skin contributes to the greater absorption of substances and increased susceptibility to irritants and allergens. Contact allergic dermatitis on the scalp is diagnosed less frequently than on other parts of the body (Zhai H. et al., 2004), and its manifestations may be insignificant, i.e., can take the form of acute and chronic itching of the scalp (Tosti A. et al., 2001). This may be due to the anatomical features of the scalp skin structure: its greater thickness and multiple pilosebaceous complexes

(Huynh M. et al., 2014). The predominance of subjective sensations in the symptomatology, the tendency of skin vessels to dilatation, and the potentiation of symptoms against the background of psycho-emotional stress indicate the involvement of the nervous system in the pathogenesis of skin hyperreactivity.

Vasodilation and degranulation of mast cells may be realized during neurogenic inflammation by releasing neurotransmitters (SP, CGRP, and VIP). Nonspecific inflammation in sensitive skin syndrome may be associated with the release of IL-1 and IL-8, prostaglandins E2 and F2, and TNFα (Reilly D.M. et al., 2000). According to some authors, one of the components of multifactorial pathogenesis may be a violation of the skin microbiome (Baldwin H.E. et al., 2017).

1.2. Diagnosis of sensitive scalp syndrome

A timely and correct diagnosis of the sensitive skin condition is important for adequate treatment. Differential diagnosis is necessary, but is complicated by the absence of vivid clinical symptoms, their small number, non-specificity and low informativeness, and the predominance of subjective symptoms.

The most common skin manifestation in sensitive skin is erythema, which may be intermittent. Irritation of sensitive scalp sometimes has a more pronounced character and is accompanied by dandruff. In such patients, the pathology can be mistakenly interpreted as seborrheic dermatitis, a disease that, in contrast to scalp sensitivity, requires a systematic approach to treatment. Careful history taking and detailed clinical examination, including dermatoscopic examination, help to suggest the presence of sensitive scalp syndrome (Lev-Tov H., Maibach H.I., 2012).

When collecting patient's history, it is important to consider:
1. Time of the pathology debut and features of its course (for example, seborrheic dermatitis emerges in puberty, and has a long wavy course with exacerbations in the autumn–winter period)
2. Subjective symptomatology (transient manifestations at the first stage and a tendency to increase the condition severity over time)
3. Skin allergic reactions to skincare, hair, and scalp care products

4. Presence of concomitant skin pathology (ichthyosis, atopic dermatitis, etc.)
5. Hypersensitivity in other parts of the body (burning, irritation of facial skin after washing, application of cosmetics, and sunscreen products)
6. Absence of the expected effect after treatment with standard antiseborrheic drugs, and refractoriness to the current therapy

Clinicians should also be attentive to the psycho-emotional condition of the patient, including consideration of the possibility of aggravated subjective complaints in dysmorphophobia.

1.3. Modern approaches to the sensitive scalp treatment

The goal of any treatment strategy for sensitive scalp syndrome is preventing the manifestations of this condition, protecting the skin from further negative effects of the environment, medications, and cosmetics, and soothing and restoring it.

The presence of sensitive skin syndrome requires a special regime of hygienic skincare and a careful selection of cosmetic products.

The components of some scalp care products (shampoos, toners, conditioners, scrubs, and peels offered by cosmetic manufacturers or prepared by patients themselves) can be excessively irritating and drying to the skin. Therefore, patients with a sensitive scalp, and especially those with signs of irritated dermatitis, should use only the necessary products with a small number of ingredients, very low concentration, and preferably free from any potentially irritating substances, sensitizers, and vasodilators.

Signs of sensitive skin can often be observed in patients with localization of any pathological process on the scalp, because of which they are forced to use topical products regularly and for a long time. Thus, it should be noted that formulations for external stimulation of hair growth often contain potentially irritating and sensitizing components: active ingredients (minoxidil), their conductors (propylene glycol), and preservatives.

The patient's understanding of the need to treat skin sensitivity will also determine the success of the overall treatment strategy.

Currently, care products for sensitive scalp are in great demand. Of particular interest to clinicians and cosmetics manufacturers are phytopreparations with soothing effects, created with traditionally used plants — chamomile, peony, and witch hazel. For example, witch hazel extract is a source of flavonoids, catechins, saponins, essential oils, choline, and tannin, which cause its vasoconstrictive, vasoconstrictive, bacteriostatic, antioxidant, and astringent actions (Trüeb R.M., 2014).

Dynamic follow-up with a specialist, especially in the first stages of sensitive scalp treatment, involves regular monitoring of the condition, which should be assessed as early as two weeks after commencing the therapy (Lev-Tov H., Maibach H.I., 2012).

Conclusion

According to surveys, about half of cosmetics consumers believe they have overly sensitive skin. In response to the market demand, cosmetics manufacturers are mastering the production of specialized products for sensitive skin, and today in almost every brand, you can find both individual products and complete lines with labels like "hypoallergenic," "for sensitive skin," etc. The presence of such products puts a lot of pressure on customers, many of whom choose them as "safer and gentler" options even if they have no skin problems.

The development of adverse reactions (itching, redness, swelling, rashes, etc.) even to a single product usually prompts a refusal of all cosmetics of the brand or the skincare professional treatments. Attempts to understand each failure are often unsuccessful. While there are several reasons for this, incorrect diagnosis is the leading cause because hypersensitive skin is not a specific pathology but a symptom complex.

Skin sensitivity syndrome is a tricky problem, as it can have different (and many) triggering factors, but there are common pathogenetic roots behind them all.

Almost always, the main link in the development of skin hypersensitivity is a violation of the integrity and increased permeability of the *stratum corneum*, which is normally a reliable barrier protecting the skin from external aggression. Therefore, it is the restoration of the barrier that must be the primary focus of all efforts to develop a strategy of care for hypersensitive skin.

Procedures that damage the skin barrier layer should be preceded and completed by measures aimed at barrier repair, antioxidant, and anti-inflammatory therapy.

An equally important factor is the increased reactivity of sensitive sensory structures of the skin, which creates prerequisites for neurogenic inflammation.

Finally, cellular damage, genetic predisposition, vascular disorders, and psychological aspects (stress and the nocebo effect) will also contribute.

Properly selected cosmetic care and therapy, considering the characteristics of the individual patient and understanding of the processes occurring in the human body, can, if not permanently solve the problem, at least provide a lasting remission and improve the quality of life — a goal worth the effort.

References

Ali S.M., Yosipovitch G. Skin pH: from basic science to basic skin care. Acta Derm Venereol. 2013; 93(3): 261–217.

Angelova-Fischer I. Irritants and skin barrier function. Curr Probl Dermatol 2016; 49: 80–89.

Angelova-Fischer I., Fischer T.W., Abels C. et al. Accelerated barrier recovery and enhancement of the barrier integrity and properties by topical application of a pH 4 vs. a pH 5·8 water-in-oil emulsion in aged skin. Br J Dermatol 2018; 179(2): 471–477.

Araviyskaya E.R. Symptom complex of sensitive skin: mechanisms of development and tactics of patient management. Clin Dermatol Venereol 2008; 5: 45–48.

Ashida Y., Denda M. Dry environment increases mast cell number and histamine content in dermis in hairless mice. Br J Dermatol 2003; 149(2): 240–247.

Aubdool A.A., Brain S.D. Neurovascular aspects of skin neurogenic inflammation. J Investig Dermatol Symp Proc 2011; 15(1): 33–39.

Baldwin H.E., Bhatia N.D., Friedman A. et al. The role of cutaneous microbiota harmony in maintaining a functional skin barrier. J Drugs Dermatol 2017; 16(1): 12–18.

Barland C.O., Zettersten E., Brown B.S. et al. Imiquimod-induced interleukin-1 alpha stimulation improves barrier homeostasis in aged murine epidermis. J Invest Dermatol 2004; 122(2): 330–336.

Baumann L. Cosmetic dermatology. Principles and practice (translated from English) Potekaev N.N. (ed). Moscow: MEDpress-Inform, 2012.

Baumbauer K.M., DeBerry J.J., Adelman P.C. et al. Keratinocytes can modulate and directly initiate nociceptive responses. ELife 2015; 4.

Behne M.J., Meyer J.W., Hanson K.M. et al. NHE1 regulates the stratum corneum permeability barrier homeostasis. Microenvironment acidification assessed with fluorescence lifetime imaging. J Biol Chem 2002; 277(49): 47399–47406.

Berardesca E. Sensitive Skin, Skin Care Products, and Cosmetics. In: Sensitive skin syndrome (2nd ed.). Honari G., Andersen R.M., Maibach H.I. (eds.). CRC Press/Taylor & Francis, 2017, p.157–159.

Berardesca E., Farage M., Maibach H. Sensitive skin: an overview. Int J Cosmet Sci 2013; 35(1): 2–8.

Bernard A., Ficheux A.S., Nedelec A.S. et al. Induction of sensitive skin and sensitive scalp by hair dyeing. Int J Eng Res Gen Sci 2016; 4: 227–239.

Bin Saif G.A., Alotaibi H.M., Alzolibani A.A. et al. Association of psychological stress with skin symptoms among medical students. Saudi Med J 2018; 39(1): 59–66.

Bizot V., Cestone E., Michelotti A., Nobile V. Improving skin hydration and age-related symptoms by oral administration of wheat glucosylceramides and di-galactosyl diglycerides: a human clinical study. Cosmetics 2017; 4(4): 37.

Blanchet-Réthoré S., Bourdès V., Mercenier A. et al. Effect of a lotion containing the heat-treated probiotic strain Lactobacillus johnsonii NCC 533 on Staphylo-coccus aureus colonization in atopic dermatitis. Clin Cosmet Investig Dermatol 2017; 10: 249–257.

Boireau-Adamezyk E., Baillet-Guffroy A., Stamatas G.N. Age-dependent changes in stratum corneum barrier function. Skin Res Technol 2014; 20(4): 409–415.

Boisnic S., Keophiphath M., Serandour A.L. et al. Polar lipids from wheat extract oil improve skin damages induced by aging: evidence from a randomized, placebo-controlled clinical trial in women and an ex vivo study on human skin explant. J Cosmet Dermatol 2019; 18(6): 2027–2036.

Bollu P.C., Sahota P. Sleep and Parkinson Disease. Mo Med 2017; 114(5): 381–386.

Boulais N., Misery L. The epidermis: a sensory tissue. Eur J Dermatol 2008; 18: 119–127.

Bourguignon L.Y., Ramez M., Gilad E. et al. Hyaluronan-CD44 interaction stimu-lates keratinocyte differentiation, lamellar body formation/secretion, and permeability barrier homeostasis. J Invest Dermatol 2006; 126(6): 1356–1365.

Bourguignon L.Y., Wong G., Xia W. et al. Selective matrix (hyaluronan) interaction with CD44 and RhoGTPase signaling promotes keratinocyte functions and overcomes age-related epidermal dysfunction. J Dermatol Sci 2013; 72(1): 32–44.

Bouvier V., Roudaut Y., Osorio N. et al. Merkel cells sense cooling with TRPM8 chan-nels. J Invest Dermatol 2018; 138(4): 946–956.

Brenaut E., Barnetche T., Le Gall-Ianotto C. et al. Triggering factors in sensitive skin from the worldwide patients' point of view: a systematic literature review and meta-analysis. J Eur Acad Dermatol Venereol 2020; 34(2): 230–238.

Buddenkotte J., Steinhoff M. Recent advances in understanding and managing ro-sacea. F1000Res 2018; 7: F1000 Faculty Rev-1885.

Byrd A.L., Belkaid Y., Segre J.A. The human skin microbiome. Nat Rev Microbiol 2018; 16(3): 143–155.

Caterina M.J. TRP channel cannabinoid receptors in skin sensation, homeostasis, and inflammation. ACS Chem Neurosci 2014; 5(11): 1107–1116.

Caterina M.J., Pang Z. TRP channels in skin biology and pathophysiology. Pharma-ceuticals (Basel) 2016; 9(4): 77.

Chan A., Mauro Th. Acidification in the epidermis and the role of secretory phos-pholipases. Dermatoendocrinol 2011; 3(2): 84–90.

Chen W., Dai R., Li L. The prevalence of self-declared sensitive skin: a systematic review and meta-analysis. J Eur Acad Dermatol Venereol 2020; 34(8): 1779–1788.

Chen Y., Fang Q., Wang Z. et al. Transient receptor potential vanilloid 4 ion channel functions as a pruriceptor in epidermal keratinocytes to evoke histaminergic itch. J Biol Chem 2016; 291: 10252–10262.

Chen Y., Lyga J. Brain-skin connection: stress, inflammation and skin aging. Inflamm Allergy Drug Targets 2014; 13(3): 177–190.

Chen Y., Yokozeki H., Katagiri K. Physiological and functional changes in the stratum corneum restored by oestrogen in an ovariectomized mice model of climacterium. Exp Dermatol 2017; 26(5): 394–401.

Choe S.J., Kim D., Kim E.J. et al. Psychological stress deteriorates skin barrier function by activating 11β-hydroxysteroid dehydrogenase 1 and the HPA Axis. Sci Rep 2018; 8(1): 6334.

Choi E.H., Man M.Q., Wang F. et al. Is endogenous glycerol a determinant of stratum corneum hydration in humans? J Invest Dermatol 2005; 125(2): 288–293.

Choi E.H., Man M.Q., Xu P. et al. Stratum corneum acidification is impaired in moderately aged human and murine skin. J Invest Dermatol 2007; 127(12): 2847–2856.

Cosgrove M.C., Franco O.H., Granger S.P. et al. Dietary nutrient intakes and skin-aging appearance among middle-aged American women. Am J Clin Nutr 2007; 86(4): 1225–1231.

Czarnowicki T., Krueger J.G., Guttman-Yassky E. Novel concepts of prevention and treatment of atopic dermatitis through barrier and immune manipulations with implications for the atopic march. J Allergy Clin Immunol 2017; 139(6): 1723–1734.

Czarnowicki T., Malajian D., Khattri S. et al. Petrolatum: barrier repair and antimicrobial responses underlying this "inert" moisturizer. J Allergy Clin Immunol 2016; 137(4): 1091–1102.

Delinasios G.J., Karbaschi M., Cooke M.S. et al. Vitamin E inhibits the UVAI induction of "light" and "dark" cyclobutane pyrimidine dimers, and oxidatively generated DNA damage, in keratinocytes. Sci Rep 2018; 8(1): 423.

Denda M., Koyama J., Hori J. et al. Age- and sex-dependent change in stratum corneum sphingolipids. Arch Dermatol Res 1993; 285(7): 415–417.

Denda M., Sokabe T., Fukumi-Tominaga T. et al. Effects of skin surface temperature on epidermal permeability barrier homeostasis. J Invest Dermatol 2007; 127: 654–659.

Denda M., Tomitaka A., Akamatsu H., Matsunaga K. Altered distribution of calcium in facial epidermis of aged adults. J Invest Dermatol 2003; 121(6): 1557–1558.

Diffey B. Sunscreen claims, risk management and consumer confidence. Int J Cosmet Sci 2020; 42(1): 1–4.

Di Marzio L., Cinque B., Cupelli F. et al. Increase of skin-ceramide levels in aged subjects following a short-term topical application of bacterial sphingomyelinase from Streptococcus thermophilus. Int J Immunopathol Pharmacol 2008; 21(1): 137–143.

Distrutti E., Monaldi L., Ricci P. et al. Gut microbiota role in irritable bowel syndrome: new therapeutic strategies. World J Gastroenterol 2016; 22(7): 2219–2241.

Do L.H.D., Azizi N., Maibach H. Sensitive skin syndrome: an update. Am J Clin Dermatol 2020; 21(3): 401–409.

Draelos Z.D. Treating the patient with multiple cosmetic product allergies. A problem-oriented approach to sensitive skin. Postgrad Med 2000; 107(7): 70–72, 75–77.

Draelos Z.D. Formulating for sensitive skin. In: Cosmeceuticals and active skin treatment. Allured Publishing, 2002. P. 78–93.

Dumas M., Sadick N.S., Noblesse E. et al. Hydrating skin by stimulating biosynthesis of aquaporins. J Drugs Dermatol 2007; 6(6 Suppl): s20–s24.

Elias P.M. Therapeutic implications of a barrier-based pathogenesis of atopic dermatitis. Ann Dermatol 2010; 22(3): 245–254.

Elias P.M. Primary role of barrier dysfunction in the pathogenesis of atopic dermatitis. Exp Dermatol 2018; 27(8): 847–851.

Emir T.L.R. (ed.) Neurobiology of TRP channels. Boca Raton (FL): CRC Press/Taylor & Francis; 2017.

Evers A.W.M., Colloca L., Blease C. et al. Implications of placebo and nocebo effects for clinical practice: expert consensus. Psychother Psychosom 2018; 87(4): 204–210.

Falcone D., Richters R.J.H., Uzunbajakava N.E. et al. Risk factors associated with sensitive skin and potential role of lifestyle habits: a cross-sectional study. Clin Exp Dermatol 2017a; 42(6): 656–658.

Falcone D., Richters R.J., Uzunbajakava N.E. et al. Sensitive skin and the influence of female hormone fluctuations: results from a cross-sectional digital survey in the Dutch population. Eur J Dermatol 2017b; 27(1): 42–48.

Fan L., Jia Y., Cui L. et al. Analysis of sensitive skin barrier function: basic indicators and sebum composition. Int J Cosmet Sci 2018; 40(2): 117–126.

Farage M.A. Does sensitive skin differ between men and women? Cutan Ocul Toxicol 2010; 29(3): 153–163.

Farage M.A., Maibach H.I. Sensitive skin: new findings yield new insights. In: Textbook of Cosmetic Dermatology. Baran R., Maibach H.I. (eds). Informa Healthcare, 2010.

Feingold K.R., Elias P.M. Role of lipids in the formation and maintenance of the cutaneous permeability barrier. Biochim Biophys Acta 2014; 1841(3): 280–294.

Fluhr J.W., Darlenski R., Lachmann N. et al. Infant epidermal skin physiology: adaptation after birth. Br J Dermatol 2012; 166(3): 483–490.

Fluhr J.W., Kao J., Jain M. et al. Generation of free fatty acids from phospholipids regulates stratum corneum acidification and integrity. J Invest Dermatol 2001; 117(1): 44–51.

Fonacier L., Noor I. Contact dermatitis and patch testing for the allergist. Ann Allergy Asthma Immunol 2018; 120(6): 592–598.

Foster M.W., Sharp R.R. Race, ethnicity, and genomics: social classifications as proxies of biological heterogeneity. Genome Res 2002; 12: 844–850.

Frankl W. To say to life "Yes!": Psychologist in a concentration camp (translated from German). M.: Alpina Non-Fiction, 2019.

Frosch P.J., Kligman A.M. A method of apraising the stinging capacity of topically applied substances. J Soc Cosmet Chem 1977; 28: 197–209.

Gallo R.L., Granstein R.D., Kang S. et al. Standard classification and pathophysiology of rosacea: The 2017 update by the National Rosacea Society Expert Committee. J Am Acad Dermatol 2018; 78(1): 148–155.

Ghadially R., Brown B.E., Sequeira-Martin S.M. et al. The aged epidermal permeability barrier. Structural, functional, and lipid biochemical abnormalities in humans and a senescent murine model. J Clin Invest 1995; 95(5): 2281–2290.

Gilhar A., Ullmann Y., Karry R. et al. Aging of human epidermis: reversal of aging changes correlates with reversal of keratinocyte fas expression and apoptosis. J Gerontol a Biol Sci Med Sci 2004; 59(5): 411–415.

Goetze S., Hiernickel C., Elsner P. Phototoxicity of doxycycline: a systematic review on clinical manifestations, frequency, cofactors, and prevention. Skin Pharmacol Physiol 2017; 30(2): 76–80.

Green B.G., Shaffer G.S. Psychophysical assessment of the chemical irritability of human skin. J Soc Cosmet Chem 1992; 43: 131–147.

Guéniche A., Bastien P., Ovigne J.M. et al. Bifidobacterium longum lysate, a new ingredient for reactive skin. Exp Dermatol 2010; 19(8): 1–8.

Guillou S., Ghabri S., Jannot C. et al. The moisturizing effect of a wheat extract food supplement on women's skin: a randomized, double-blind placebo-controlled trial. Int J Cosmet Sci 2011; 33(2): 138–143.

Hachem J.P., Crumrine D., Fluhr J. et al. pH directly regulates epidermal permeability barrier homeostasis, and stratum corneum integrity/cohesion. J Invest Dermatol 2003; 121(2): 345–353.

Hachem J.P., Roelandt T., Schürer N. et al. Acute acidification of stratum corneum membrane domains using polyhydroxyl acids improves lipid processing and inhibits degradation of corneodesmosomes. J Invest Dermatol 2010; 130(2): 500–510.

Hanson K.M., Behne M.J., Barry N.P. et al. Two-photon fluorescence lifetime imaging of the skin stratum corneum pH gradient. Biophys J 2002; 83(3): 1682–1590

Hanifin J.M., Rajka G. Diagnostic features of atopic dermatitis. Acta Dermato-Venereol 1980; 60(92): 44–47.

Hara M., Ma T., Verkman A.S. Selectively reduced glycerol in skin of aquaporin-3-deficient mice may account for impaired skin hydration, elasticity, and barrier recovery. J Biol Chem 2002; 277(48): 46616–46621.

Hettwer S., Bänziger S., Suter B. et al. Grifolin derivatives from Albatrellus ovinus as TRPV1 receptor blockers for cosmetic applications. Int J Cosmet Sci 2017; 39(4): 379–385.

Hillion M., Mijouin L., Jaouen T. et al. Comparative study of normal and sensitive skin aerobic bacterial populations. Microbiologyopen 2013; 2(6): 953–961.

Hjell L., Ziegler D. Theories of personality (3rd ed.). SPb: Piter, 2009.

Hong J.Y., Park S.J., Seo S.J. et al. Oily sensitive skin: a review of management options. J Cosmet Dermatol 2020 May; 19(5): 1016–1020.

Hu L., Mauro T.M., Dang E. et al. Epidermal dysfunction leads to an age-associated increase in levels of serum inflammatory cytokines. J Invest Dermatol 2017; 137(6): 1277–1285.

Huang H.C., Chang T.M. Ceramide 1 and ceramide 3 act synergistically on skin hydration and the transepidermal water loss of sodium lauryl sulfate-irritated skin. Int J Dermatol 2008; 47(8): 812–819.

Huang L.N., Zhong Y.P., Liu D. et al. Adverse cutaneous reactions to skin care products on the face vary with age, but not with sex. Contact Dermat 2018; 79(6): 365–369.

Huang Y.S., Huang W.C., Li C.W., Chuang L.T. Eicosadienoic acid differentially modulates production of pro-inflammatory modulators in murine macrophages. Mol Cell Biochem 2011; 358(1–2): 85–94.

Huet F., Dion A., Batardière A. et al. Sensitive skin can be small fbre neuropathy: results from a case-control quantitative sensory testing study. Br J Dermatol 2018; 179(5): 1157–1162.

Huynh M., Sheehan M.P., Chung M. et al. Scalp. In: Clinical Handbook of Contact Dermatitis. Diagnosis and Management by Body Region. Lewallen R., Clark A., Feldman S.R. (eds): CRC Press, 2014, pp. 6–12.

Igawa S., Di Nardo A. Skin microbiome and mast cells. Transl Res 2017; 184: 68–76.

Ikarashi N., Kon R., Kaneko M. et al. Relationship between aging-related skin dryness and aquaporins. Int J Mol Sci 2017; 18(7): E1559.

Imokawa G., Abe A., Jin K. et al. Decreased level of ceramides in stratum corneum of atopic dermatitis: an etiologic factor in atopic dry skin? J Invest Dermatol 1991; 96(4): 523–526.

Inamadar A.C., Palit A. Sensitive skin: An overview. Indian J Dermatol Venereol Leprol 2013; 79: 9–16.

Jack A.R., Norris P.L., Storrs F.J. Allergic contact dermatitis to plant extracts in cosmetics. Semin Cutan Med Surg 2013; 32(3): 140–146.

Jang H., Matsuda A., Jung K. et al. Skin pH Is the master switch of kallikrein 5-mediated skin barrier destruction in a murine atopic dermatitis model. J Invest Dermatol 2016; 136(1): 127–135.

Jiang B., Cui L., Zi Y. et al. Skin surface lipid differences in sensitive skin caused by psychological stress and distinguished by support vector machine. J Cosmet Dermatol 2019; 18(4): 1121–1127.

Jiang W.C., Zhang H., Xu Y. et al. Cutaneous vessel features of sensitive skin and its underlying functions. Skin Res Technol 2020; 26(3): 431–437.

Jiang Y.J., Lu B., Crumrine D. et al. IL-1alpha accelerates stratum corneum formation and improves permeability barrier homeostasis during murine fetal development. J Dermatol Sci 2009; 54(2): 88–98.

Jinnestål C.L., Belfrage E., Bäck O. et al. Skin barrier impairment correlates with cutaneous Staphylococcus aureus colonization and sensitization to skin-associated microbial antigens in adult patients with atopic dermatitis. Int J Dermatol 2014; 53(1): 27–33.

Kail-Goryachkina M.V., Belousova T.A. Syndrome of sensitive skin in the practice of a dermatologist. Consilium Medicum. Dermatologia 2016; 1: 22–26.

Kao J.S., Fluhr J.W., Man M.Q. et al. Short-term glucocorticoid treatment compromises both permeability barrier homeostasis and stratum corneum integrity: inhibition of epidermal lipid synthesis accounts for functional abnormalities. J Invest Dermatol 2003; 120(3): 456–464.

Karlsson C., Andersson M.L., Collin M. et al. SufA — a novel subtilisin-like serine proteinase of Finegoldia magna. Microbiology (Reading). 2007; 153(Pt 12): 4208–4218.

Keum H.L., Kim H., Kim H.J. et al. Structures of the skin microbiome and mycobiome depending on skin sensitivity. Microorganisms 2020; 8(7): 1032.

Khandpur S., Porter R.M., Boulton S.J. et al. Drug-induced photosensitivity: new insights into pathomechanisms and clinical variation through basic and applied science. Br J Dermatol 2017; 176(4): 902–909.

Kida N., Sokabe T., Kashio M. Importance of transient receptor potential vanilloid 4 (TRPV4) in epidermal barrier function in human skin keratinocytes. Pflugers Arch 2012; 463: 715–725.

Kilic A., Masur C., Reich H. et al. Skin acidification with a water-in-oil emulsion (pH 4) restores disrupted epidermal barrier and improves structure of lipid lamellae in the elderly. J Dermatol 2019; 46(6): 457–465.

Kim E.J., Lee D.H., Kim Y.K. et al. Decreased ATP synthesis and lower pH may lead to abnormal muscle contraction and skin sensitivity in human skin. J Dermatol Sci 2014; 76(3): 214–221.

Kim E.J., Lee D.H., Kim Y.K. et al. Adiponectin deficiency contributes to sensitivity in human skin. J Invest Dermatol 2015; 135: 2331–2334.

Kim H.S., Yosipovitch G. The skin microbiota and itch: is there a link? J Clin Med 2020; 9(4): 1190.

Kinn P.M., Holdren G.O., Westermeyer B.A. et al. Age-dependent variation in cytokines, chemokines, and biologic analytes rinsed from the surface of healthy human skin. Sci Rep 2015; 5: 10472.

Kiousi D.E., Karapetsas A., Karolidou K. et al. Probiotics in extraintestinal diseases: current trends and new directions. Nutrients 2019; 11(4): 788.

Kligman A.M. Human models for characterizing "sensitive skin." Cosmet Dermatol 2001; 14: 15–19.

Kligman A.M., Sadiq I., Zhen Y. et al. Experimental studies on the nature of sensitive skin. Skin Res Technol 2006; 12(4): 217–222.

Korting H.C., Hübner K., Greiner K., et al. Differences in the skin surface pH and bacterial microflora due to the long-term application of synthetic detergent preparations of pH 5.5 and pH 7.0. Results of a crossover trial in healthy volunteers. Acta Derm Venereol 1990; 70(5): 429–431.

Krien P.M., Kermici M. Evidence for the existence of a self-regulated enzymatic process within the human stratum corneum -an unexpected role for urocanic acid. J Invest Dermatol 2000; 115(3): 414–420.

Kwa M., Welty L.J., Xu S. Adverse events reported to the US Food and Drug Administration for cosmetics and personal care products. JAMA Intern Med 2017; 177(8): 1202–1204.

Lee H.J., Lee N.R., Kim B.K. et al. Acidification of stratum corneum prevents the progression from atopic dermatitis to respiratory allergy. Exp Dermatol 2017; 26(1): 66–72.

Lee Y.S., Yi J.S., Lim H.R. et al. Phototoxicity evaluation of pharmaceutical substances with a reactive oxygen species assay using ultraviolet A. Toxicol Res 2017; 33(1): 43–48.

Lev-Tov H., Maibach H.I. The sensitive skin syndrome. Indian J Dermatol 2012; 57(6): 419–423.

Li J., Tang H., Hu X. et al. Aquaporin-3 gene and protein expression in sun-protected human skin decreases with skin ageing. Australas J Dermatol 2010; 51(2): 106–112.

Liccardi G., Senna G., Russo M. et al. Evaluation of the nocebo effect during oral challenge in patients with adverse drug reactions. J Investig Allergol Clin Immunol 2004; 14: 104–107.

Lin T.K., Man M.Q., Santiago J.L. et al. Topical antihistamines display potent anti-inflammatory activity linked in part to enhanced permeability barrier function. J Invest Dermatol 2013; 133(2): 469–478.

Liu T., Gao Y.J., Ji R.R. Emerging role of Toll-like receptors in the control of pain and itch. Neurosci Bull 2012; 28(2): 131–144.

Luebberding S., Krueger N., Kerscher M. Age-related changes in skin barrier function — quantitative evaluation of 150 female subjects. Int J Cosmet Sci 2013a; 35(2): 183–190.

Luebberding S., Krueger N., Kerscher M. Skin physiology in men and women: in vivo evaluation of 300 people including TEWL, SC hydration, sebum content and skin surface pH. Int J Cosmet Sci 2013b; 35(5): 477–483.

Ma Z.S. Testing the Anna Karenina principle in human microbiome-associated diseases. iScience 2020; 23(4): 101007.

Maibach H.I. The cosmetic intolerance syndrome. Ear Nose Throat J 1987; 66(1): 29–33.

Man M.Q., Choi E.H., Schmuth M. et al. Basis for improved permeability barrier homeostasis induced by PPAR and LXR activators: liposensors stimulate lipid synthesis, lamellar body secretion, and post-secretory lipid processing. J Invest Dermatol 2006; 126(2): 386–392.

Man M.Q., Elias P.M. Stratum corneum hydration regulates key epidermal function and serves as an indicator and contributor to other conditions. J Eur Acad Dermatol Venereol 2019; 33(1): 15–16.

Man M.Q., Feingold K.R., Elias P.M. Exogenous lipids influence permeability barrier recovery in acetone-treated murine skin. Arch Dermatol 1993; 129(6): 728–738.

Man M.Q., Feingold K.R., Jain M., Elias P.M. Extracellular processing of phospholipids is required for permeability barrier homeostasis. J Lipid Res 1995; 36(9): 1925–1935.

Man M.Q., Feingold K.R., Thornfeldt C.R., Elias P.M. Optimization of physiological lipid mixtures for barrier repair. J Invest Dermatol 1996; 106(5): 1096–1101.

Man M.Q., Xin S.J., Song S.P. et al. Variation of skin surface pH, sebum content and stratum corneum hydration with age and gender in a large Chinese population. Skin Pharmacol Physiol 2009; 22(4): 190–199.

Marek-Jozefowicz L., Nedoszytko B., Grochocka M. et al. Molecular mechanisms of neurogenic inflammation of the skin. Int J Mol Sci. 2023; 24(5): 5001.

Marriott M., Holmes J., Peters L. et al. The complex problem of sensitive skin. Contact Derm 2005; 53: 93–99.

Micallef L., Belaubre F., Pinon A. et al. Effects of extracellular calcium on the growth-differentiation switch in immortalized keratinocyte HaCaT cells compared with normal human keratinocytes. Exp Dermatol 2009; 18(2): 143–151.

Mills O.H., Berger R.S. Defining the susceptibility of acne-prone and sensitive skin populations to extrinsic factors. Dermatol Clin 1991; 1: 93–98.

Miri A., Beiki H., Sarani M. Cerium oxide nanoparticles: biosynthesis, cytotoxic and UV protection. Preprints 2020, 2020070487.

Misery L. Neuropsychiatric factors in sensitive skin. Clin Dermatol 2017; 35(3): 281–284.

Misery L., Boussetta S., Nocera T. et al. Sensitive skin in Europe. J Eur Acad Dermatol Venereol 2009; 23(4): 376–381.

Misery L., Dutray S., Chastaing M. et al. Psychogenic itch. Transl Psychiatry 2018; 8(1): 52.

Misery L., Jean-Decoster C., Mery S. et al. A new ten-item questionnaire for assessing sensitive skin: the Sensitive Scale-10. Acta Derm Venereol 2014; 94(6): 635–639.

Misery L., Sibaud V., Ambronati M. et al. Sensitive scalp: does this condition exist? An epidemiological study. Contact Dermatitis 2008; 58(4): 234–238.

Misery L., Sibaud V., Merial-Kieny C. et al. Sensitive skin in the American population: prevalence, clinical data, and role of the dermatologist. Int J Dermatol 2011; 50(8): 961–967.

Misery L., Ständer S., Szepietowski J.C. et al. Definition of sensitive skin: an expert position paper from the special interest group on sensitive skin of the International Forum for the Study of Itch. Acta Derm Venereol 2017; 97: 4–6.

Misery L., Weisshaar E., Brenaut E. et al Special Interest Group on sensitive skin of the International Forum for the Study of Itch (ISFI). Pathophysiology and management of sensitive skin: position paper from the special interest group on sensitive skin of the International Forum for the Study of Itch (IFSI). J Eur Acad Dermatol Venereol 2020a; 34(2): 222–229.

Moehring F., Cowie A.M., Menzel A.D. et al. Keratinocytes mediate innocuous and noxious touch via ATP-P2X4 signaling. ELife 2018; 7.

Moore C., Cevikbas F., Pasolli H.A. et al. UVB radiation generates sunburn pain and affects skin by activating epidermal TRPV4 ion channels and triggering endothelin-1 signaling. Proc Natl Acad Sci USA 2013; 110: E3225–3234.

Mottin V.H.M., Suyenaga E.S. An approach on the potential use of probiotics in the treatment of skin conditions: acne and atopic dermatitis. Int J Dermatol 2018; 57(12): 1425–1432.

Muizzuddin N., Maher W., Sullivan M. et al. Physiological effect of a probiotic on skin. J Cosmet Sci 2012; 63(6): 385–395.

Negulescu M., Zerdoud S., Boulinguez S. et al. Development of photoonycholysis with vandetanib therapy. Skin Appendage Disord 2017; 2(3–4): 146–151.

Nikolaeva N.N. The role of the patient's emotional state in the development of undesirable phenomena and complications in the practice of a cosmetologist. Injection Methods Cosmetol 2017; 4: 24–28.

Novitskaya N.N. Psychotherapy in the treatment of patients with psoriasis. Cosm & Med 2015; 4: 46–49.

Onoue S., Seto Y., Sato H. et al. Chemical photoallergy: photobiochemical mechanisms, classification, and risk assessments. J Dermatol Sci 2017; 85(1): 4–11.

Pang Z., Sakamoto T., Tiwari V. et al. Selective keratinocyte stimulation is sufficient to evoke nociception in mice. Pain 2015; 156: 656–665.

Park M.E., Zippin J.H. Allergic contact dermatitis to cosmetics. Dermatol Clin 2014; 32(1): 1–11.

Parrado C., Mercado-Saenz S., Perez-Davo A. et al. Environmental stressors on skin aging. Mechanistic Insights. Front Pharmacol 2019; 10: 759.

Páyer E., Szabó-Papp J., Ambrus L. et al. Beyond the physico-chemical barrier: glycerol and xylitol markedly yet differentially alter gene expression profiles and modify signalling pathways in human epidermal keratinocytes. Exp Dermatol 2018; 27(3): 280–284.

Prakash A.V., Davis M.D. Contact dermatitis in older adults: a review of the literature. Am J Clin Dermatol 2010; 11(6): 373–381.

Prescott S.L., Larcombe D.L., Logan A.C. et al. The skin microbiome: impact of modern environments on skin ecology, barrier integrity, and systemic immune programming. J World Allergy Organ 2017; 10(1): 29.

Querleux B., Dauchot K., Jourdain R. et al. Neural basis of sensitive skin: an fMRI study. Skin Res Technol 2008; 14(4): 454–461.

Rebora A., Semino M.T., Guarrera M. Trichodynia. Dermatol 1996; 192(3): 292–293.

Reilly D.M., Parslew R., Sharpe G.R. et al. Inflammatory mediators in normal, sensitive and diseased skintypes. Acta Derm Venereol 2000; 80(3): 171–174.

Richters R.J.H., Uzunbajakava N.E., Hendriks J.C.M. et al. A model for perception-based identification of sensitive skin. J Eur Acad Dermatol Venereol 2017; 31: 267–273.

Rinnerthaler M., Duschl J., Steinbacher P. et al. Age-related changes in the composition of the cornified envelope in human skin. Exp Dermatol 2013; 22(5): 329–335.

Rippke F., Berardesca E., Weber T.M. pH and microbial Infections. Curr Probl Dermatol 2018; 54: 87–94.

Rogers J., Harding C., Mayo A. et al. Stratum corneum lipids: the effect of ageing and the seasons. Arch Dermatol Res 1996; 288(12): 765–770.

Roussaki-Schulze A.V., Zafriou E., Nikoulis D. et al. Objective biophysical fndings in patients with sensitive skin. Drugs Exp Clin Res 2005; 31(Suppl): 17–24.

Saint-Martory C., Roguedas-Contios A.M., Sibaud V. et al. Sensitive skin is not limited to the face. Br J Dermatol 2008; 158(1): 130–133.

Sann H., Pierau F.K. Efferent functions of C-fiber nociceptors. Z Rheumatol 1998; 57(Suppl 2): 8–13.

Scharschmidt T.C., Man M.Q., Hatano Y. et al. Filaggrin deficiency confers a paracellular barrier abnormality that reduces inflammatory thresholds to irritants and haptens. J Allergy Clin Immunol 2009; 124(3): 496–506, 506.e1–6.

Scheenstra M.R., van Harten R.M., Veldhuizen E.J.A. et al. Cathelicidins modulate TLR-activation and inflammation. Front Immunol 2020; 11: 1137.

Schrader A., Siefken W., Kueper T. et al. Effects of glyceryl glucoside on AQP3 expression, barrier function and hydration of human skin. Skin Pharmacol Physiol 2012; 25(4): 192–199.

Schreml S., Zeller V., Meier R.J. et al. Impact of age and body site on adult female skin surface pH. Dermatology 2012; 224(1): 66–71.

Seidenari S., Francomano M., Mantavoni L. Baseline biophysical parameters in subjects with sensitive skin. Contact Dermatitis 1998; 38(6): 311–315.

Seite S., Misery L. Skin sensitivity and skin microbiota: is there a link? Exp Dermatol 2018; 27(9): 1061–1064.

Simion F.A., Rau A.H. Sensitive skin. In: Cosmeceuticals and active skin treatment. Allured Publishing 2002; 67–77.

Simion F.A., Rhein L.D., Morrison B.M. et al. Self-perceived sensory responses to soap and synthetic detergent bars correlate with clinical signs of irritation. J Am Acad Dermatol 1995; 32(2 Pt 1): 205–211.

Snatchfold J. Cutaneous acceptability of a moisturizing cream in subjects with sensitive skin. J Cosmet Dermatol 2019; 18(1): 226–229.

Soeur J., Belaïdi J.P., Chollet C. et al. Photo-pollution stress in skin: traces of pollutants (PAH and particulate matter) impair redox homeostasis in keratinocytes exposed to UVA1. J Dermatol Sci 2017; 86(2): 162–169.

Sonbol H., Brenaut E., Nowak E. et al. Efficacy and tolerability of phototherapy with light-emitting diodes for sensitive skin: a pilot study. Front Med (Lausanne). 2020; 7: 35.

Storozhuk M.V., Zholos A.V. TRP channels as novel targets for endogenous ligands: focus on endocannabinoids and nociceptive signalling. Curr Neuropharmacol 2018; 16(2): 137–150.

Stumpf A., Zerey V., Heuft G. et al. Itch perception and skin reactions as modulated by verbal suggestions: role of participant's and investigator's sex. Acta Derm Venereol 2016; 96: 619–623.

Sun C.Y., Cao Z., Zhang X.J. et al. Cascade-amplifying synergistic effects of chemo-photodynamic therapy using ROS-responsive polymeric nanocarriers. Theranostics 2018; 8(11): 2939–2953.

Szepietowski J., Reich A. Pruritus and psoriasis. Br J Dermatol 2004; 151(6): 1284.

Taïeb C., Misery L. Sensitive skin: a review of prevalence worldwide. In: Sensitive skin syndrome (2nd ed.). Honari G., Andersen R.M., Maibach H.I. (eds.). CRC Press/Taylor & Francis, 2017, p. 233.

Takahashi M., Tezuka T. The content of free amino acids in the stratum corneum is increased in senile xerosis. Arch Dermatol Res 2004; 295(10): 448–452.

Talagas M., Lebonvallet N., Leschiera R. et al. What about physical contacts between epidermal keratinocytes and sensory neurons? Exp Dermatol 2018; 27(1): 9–13.

Talagas M., Misery L. Role of keratinocytes in sensitive skin. Front Med 2019; 6: 108.

Tan C.H., Rasool S., Johnston G.A. Contact dermatitis: allergic and irritant. Clin Dermatol 2014; 32(1): 116–124.

Tan J., Berg M. Rosacea: current state of epidemiology. J Am Acad Dermatol 2013; 69(6 Suppl 1): S27–S35.

Tanei R., Hasegawa Y. Atopic dermatitis in older adults: a viewpoint from geriatric dermatology. Geriatr Gerontol Int 2016; 16(Suppl 1): 75–86.

Thornton M.J. Estrogens and aging skin. Dermatoendocrinol 2013; 5(2): 264–270.

Tiganescu A., Hupe M., Uchida Y. et al. Topical 11β-hydroxysteroid dehydrogenase type 1 inhibition corrects cutaneous features of systemic glucocorticoid excess in female mice. Endocrinol 2018; 159(1): 547–556.

Tiganescu A., Tahrani A.A., Morgan S.A. et al. 11β-Hydroxysteroid dehydrogenase blockade prevents age-induced skin structure and function defects. J Clin Invest 2013; 123(7): 3051–3060.

Tiganescu A., Walker E.A., Hardy R.S. et al. Localization, age- and site-dependent expression, and regulation of 11β-hydroxysteroid dehydrogenase type 1 in skin. J Invest Dermatol 2011; 131(1): 30–36.

Tomlinson J.W., Walker E.A., Bujalska I.J. et al. 11beta-hydroxysteroid dehydrogenase type 1: a tissue-specific regulator of glucocorticoid response. Endocr Rev 2004; 25(5): 831–866.

Tosti A., Piraccini B.M., van Neste D.J. Telogen effluvium after allergic contact dermatitis of the scalp. Arch Dermatol 2001; 137(2): 187–190.

Trüeb R.M. North American Virginian Witch Hazel (Hamamelis virginiana): based scalp care and protection for sensitive scalp, red scalp, and scalp burn-out. Int J Trichol 2014; 6(3): 100–103.

Valdes-Rodriguez R., Stull C., Yosipovitch G. Chronic pruritus in the elderly: pathophysiology, diagnosis and management. Drugs Aging 2015; 32(3): 201–215.

Vaughn A.R., Clark A.K., Sivamani R.K., Shi V.Y. Natural oils for skin-barrier repair: ancient compounds now backed by modern science. Am J Clin Dermatol 2018; 19(1): 103–117.

Vávrová K., Henkes D., Strüver K. et al. Filaggrin deficiency leads to impaired lipid profile and altered acidification pathways in a 3D skin construct. J Invest Dermatol 2014; 134(3): 746–753.

Wang X., Su Y., Zheng B. et al. Gender-related characterization of sensitive skin in normal young Chinese. J Cosmet Dermatol 2020; 19(5): 1137–1142.

Wang Z., Man M.Q., Li T. et al. Aging-associated alterations in epidermal function and their clinical significance. Aging 2020; 12(6): 5551–5565.

Wanke I., Skabytska Y., Kraft B. et al. Staphylococcus aureus skin colonization is promoted by barrier disruption and leads to local inflammation. Exp Dermatol 2013; 22(2): 153–155.

Wilkin J., Dahl M., Detmar M. et al. Standard classification system of rosacea: report of the National Rosacea Society Expert Committee on the Classification and Staging of Rosacea. J Am Acad Dermatol 2002; 46: 584–587.

Willimann B., Trüeb R.M. Hair pain (trichodynia): frequency and relationship to hair loss and patient gender. Dermatol 2002; 205(4): 374–377.

Willis C.M., Shaw S., De Lacharrière O. et al. Sensitive skin: an epidemiological study. Br J Dermatol 2001; 145(2): 258–263.

Yamamoto A., Serizawa S., Ito M., Sato Y. Effect of aging on sebaceous gland activity and on the fatty acid composition of wax esters. J Invest Dermatol 1987; 89(5): 507–512.

Yang L., Lyu L., Wu W. et al. Genome-wide identifcation of long non-coding RNA and mRNA profiling using RNA sequencing in subjects with sensitive skin. Oncotarget 2017; 8(70): 114894–114910.

Yang L., Mao-Q.M., Taljebini M. et al. Topical stratum corneum lipids accelerate barrier repair after tape stripping, solvent treatment and some but not all types of detergent treatment. Br J Dermatol 1995; 133(5): 679–685.

Ye J., Garg A., Calhoun C. et al. Alterations in cytokine regulation in aged epidermis: implications for permeability barrier homeostasis and inflammation. I. IL-1 gene family. Exp Dermatol 2002; 11(3): 209–216.

Ye L., Mauro T.M., Dang E. et al. Topical applications of an emollient reduce circulating pro-inflammatory cytokine levels in chronically aged humans: a pilot clinical study. J Eur Acad Dermatol Venereol 2019; 33(11): 2197–2201.

Yiallouris A., Tsioutis C., Agapidaki E. et al. Adrenal aging and its implications on stress responsiveness in humans. Front Endocrinol 2019; 10: 54.

Yokota T., Matsumoto M., Sakamaki T. Classification of sensitive skin and development of treatment system appropriate for each group. IFSCC Magazine 2003; 6: 303–307.

Young A.R., Claveau J., Rossi A.B. Ultraviolet radiation and the skin: photobiology and sunscreen photoprotection. J Am Acad Dermatol 2017; 76(3S1): 100–109.

Yuan C., Ma Y., Wang Y. et al. Rosacea is associated with conjoined interactions between physical barrier of the skin and microorganisms: a pilot study. J Clin Lab Anal 2020; 34(9): e23363.

Zettersten E.M., Ghadially R., Feingold K.R. et al. Optimal ratios of topical stratum corneum lipids improve barrier recovery in chronologically aged skin. J Am Acad Dermatol 1997; 37(3 Pt 1): 403–408.

Zha W.F., Song W.M., Ai J.J. et al. Mobile connected dermatoscope and confocal laser scanning microscope: a useful combination applied in facial simple sensitive skin. Int J Cosmet Sci 2012; 34: 318–321.

Zhai H., Fautz R., Fuchs A. et al. Human scalp irritation compared to that of the arm and back. Contact Dermatitis 2004; 51(4): 196–200.

Zlotogorski A. Distribution of skin surface pH on the forehead and cheek of adults. Arch Dermatol Res 1987; 279(6): 398–401.